Complex Care in Nursing

Sara Miller McCune founded SAGE Publishing in 1965 to support the dissemination of usable knowledge and educate a global community. SAGE publishes more than 1000 journals and over 800 new books each year, spanning a wide range of subject areas. Our growing selection of library products includes archives, data, case studies and video. SAGE remains majority owned by our founder and after her lifetime will become owned by a charitable trust that secures the company's continued independence.

Los Angeles | London | New Delhi | Singapore | Washington DC | Melbourne

Complex Care in Nursing

Sally-Anne Wherry
Nikki Buck

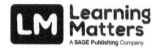

Learning Matters
A SAGE Publishing Company
1 Oliver's Yard
55 City Road
London EC1Y 1SP

SAGE Publications Inc.
2455 Teller Road
Thousand Oaks, California 91320

SAGE Publications India Pvt Ltd
B 1/I 1 Mohan Cooperative Industrial Area
Mathura Road
New Delhi 110 044

SAGE Publications Asia-Pacific Pte Ltd
3 Church Street
#10-04 Samsung Hub
Singapore 049483

Editor: Laura Walmsley
Development editor: Sarah Turpie
Senior project editor: Chris Marke
Marketing manager: Ruslana Khatagova
Cover design: Sheila Tong
Typeset by: C&M Digitals (P) Ltd, Chennai, India
Printed in the UK

Library of Congress Control Number: 2022943271

British Library Cataloguing in Publication Data

A catalogue record for this book is available from the
British Library

ISBN 978-1-5297-6434-5
ISBN 978-1-5297-6435-2 (pbk)

At SAGE we take sustainability seriously. Most of our products are printed in the UK using responsibly sourced
papers and boards. When we print overseas we ensure sustainable papers are used as measured by the PREPS
grading system. We undertake an annual audit to monitor our sustainability.

Contents

TRANSFORMING NURSING PRACTICE

Transforming Nursing Practice is a series tailor made for pre-registration student nurses. Each book in the series is:

- Affordable
- Mapped to the NMC Standards of proficiency for registered nurses
- Full of active learning features
- Focused on applying theory to practice

Each book addresses a core topic and they have been carefully developed to be simple to use, quick to read and written in clear language.

An invaluable series of books that explicitly relates to the NMC standards. Each book covers a different topic that students need to explore in order to develop into a qualified nurse... I would recommend this series to all Pre-Registered nursing students whatever their field or year of study.

LINDA ROBSON,
Senior Lecturer at Edge Hill University

Many titles in the series are on our recommended reading list and for good reason - the content is up to date and easy to read. These are the books that actually get used beyond training and into your nursing career.

EMMA LYDON,
Adult Student Nursing

ABOUT THE SERIES EDITORS

DR MOOI STANDING is an Independent Nursing Consultant (UK and International) and is responsible for the core knowledge, adult nursing and personal and professional learning skills titles. She is an experienced NMC Quality Assurance Reviewer of educational programmes and a Professional Regulator Panellist on the NMC Practice Committee. Mooi is also Board member of Special Olympics Malaysia, enabling people with intellectual disabilities to participate in sports and athletics nationally and internationally.

DR SANDRA WALKER is a Clinical Academic in Mental Health working between Southern Health Trust and the University of Southampton and responsible for the mental health nursing titles. She is a Qualified Mental Health Nurse with a wide range of clinical experience spanning more than 25 years.

BESTSELLING TEXTBOOKS

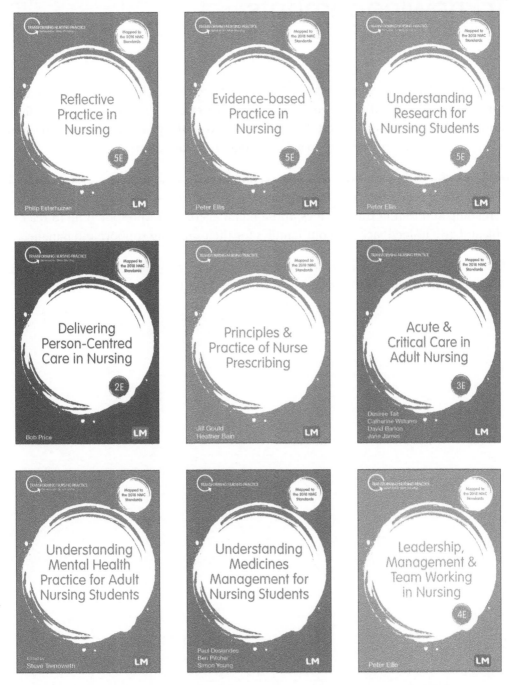

Acknowledgements

This book reflects the collective knowledge of many people, including our experts by experience and clinical colleagues without whose efforts this work would be significantly weaker and less rounded. It reflects the work of five nurses working together during a pandemic, and we want to acknowledge that team effort.

It is important to acknowledge those who contribute to our work and so we would like to thank the experts by experience who gave us their time and energy, our students for reading and testing the activities, those members of staff who took time to read the book and give us feedback, and our families for their ongoing support and patience.

The team behind any book includes the editors and proof-readers, without whom this book would be considerably less polished and connected.

About the Authors

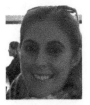 **Sally-Anne Wherry** (she/her) is a senior lecturer in Gloucestershire, where she teaches undergraduates and postgraduates. A specialist Parkinson and movement disorder nurse, she now teaches nurses in topics such as ethics, research, shared decision-making, long-term and complex conditions, and prescribing. She has focused on self-management and shared decision-making in her research and is currently working on a PhD around intergenerational trauma.

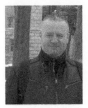 **Nikki Buck** (she/her) is a senior lecturer in Gloucestershire, where she teaches undergraduates. She is an experienced neonatal intensive care nurse and teaches nurses with a specialist interest in anatomy and physiology.

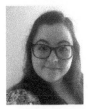 **Nick Preddy** (he/him) qualified as a Learning Disabilities Nurse in 1993 and has worked across a range of services for people with learning disabilities with an interest in autism and profound and multiple disabilities. Nick's strongest passion in teaching is the ethics and values-base involved in Learning Disabilities Nursing and how nurses can lead and promote values-based services. Nick is a strong advocate for the involvement of experts by experience in the development, delivery and evaluation of educational and works in partnership with professionals in Zagreb, Croatia to provide students with an overseas field trip experience.

 Sam Greedy (she/her) is a lecturer in Gloucestershire, after a career working as a specialist nurse with people with learning disabilities and complex mental health needs. She has worked as a part of a community learning disability team, supporting people with complex behavioural presentations. She has also worked in a specialist CAMHS service, supporting children and young people with a learning disability and autism. Sam's key interests are in complex behaviour management and family-centred care.

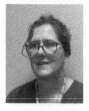

Eleri Jones (she/her) is a mental health nurse prescriber, working in primary care in Gloucestershire. She works with people with varying degrees of distress and mental illness.

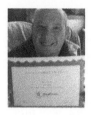

Mark Smith is an expert by experience with a diagnosis of 'mild learning disabilities'. He works as a visiting lecturer at two universities teaching across a variety of health and social care programmes.

Introduction

This book is a collaboration between experts by experience, clinicians and academics. The aim is to introduce you to living with complex needs, through the lens of patients and the experts in the field. We hope it aids you in developing reflective, holistic practice and understanding some of the forces that create the situations people are living in.

Chapter 1 will talk about the definition and statistics we will be using, as well as introducing you to the people you will meet in this book, including our experts by experience and healthcare teams. We will discuss the impact of living with a complex need, including the additional costs.

Chapter 2 will provide you with the context of the discussions in the later chapters. It will talk about the powers that work on people living with complex needs, including sociological, political, psychological and biological drives. We'll explore practical issues around medication and concordance. We'll discuss events that might drive some of the changes to policy.

Chapter 3 explores the impact of socioeconomics in complex care such as living on benefits, including the impact of appeals. We'll introduce you to the Vimes theory of socioeconomics, and the disability price tag. The chapter will (hopefully) give you insight into how we measure cost-effectiveness in the NHS, the quality-adjusted life year and health disparities.

Chapter 4 explores the nursing process, assessing your patients and the management of your own emotions. We'll talk about the collaboration that can exist between the person living with complexity and the healthcare team. We'll discuss different measurements that are used in this area.

Chapter 5 explores the multidisciplinary team a little more, and different models of care. It will discuss the House of Care model in more depth, including an implementation of it and the critiques.

Chapter 6 discusses shared decision-making, a vital part of caring for someone with complex needs. We'll go into more depth on three models: the three-talk mode, the interprofessional SDM model and the Ottawa Decision Support Framework. We'll talk about capacity and consent.

Chapter 7 focuses on those living with mental health needs, the impact of those on physical health and the social and political determinants which impacts this group. We'll talk about trauma-informed care, communication and ethics. We will discuss capacity and consent. We will explore the funding within the NHS and access to support needs. We will investigate several models of care.

Chapter 8 provides some more views on living with complex needs as an adult. We will explore energy management, team working, communication and sexuality.

Chapter 9 looks at the needs of people with learning disabilities. It will provide definitions, labels and give you some understanding of autism. It will explore sensory issues, communication, behaviour and comorbidities. It will provide you with some techniques that your patients may be using.

Chapter 10 explores the experience of the child living with complex needs, and their family. It will discuss capacity and consent, including the Fraser guidelines and Gillick competence. It will explore the models of care that are common in young people and children's health services.

NMC's Standards of Proficiency for Registered Nurses

The Nursing and Midwifery Council (NMC) has Standards of Proficiency that must be met by applicants to different parts of the nursing and midwifery register. These standards are what they deem as being necessary for the delivery of safe, effective nursing and midwifery practice.

This book includes the latest standards for 2018 onwards, taken from *Future Nurse: Standards of Proficiency for Registered Nurses* (Nursing and Midwifery Council, 2018).

Learning features

Textbooks are not easy reading, but throughout this text you will find activities and case studies which we hope will help you to pause and place the information you have read into the context of a person or your practice. You will need to rely on your study skills to get the best of this book. We have not focused on conditions, and you are expected to go and find more information that you feel you need.

The activities are designed to help you understand the world of the person living with complex needs. Some of them will ask you to reflect, while others will require some critical thinking; these are vital skills you will use in your practice. During your time as a nurse, you will be expected to plan care with people, and some activities are aimed at helping you to understand some of the key aspects of this role.

All the activities ask you to pause in your reading, to consider the issues we have raised and perhaps go and find more information or apply your own practice to the question. There are some sample answers at the end of chapters, but we suggest that you finish the activity yourself before looking at them to get the most of out of the work. As you likely have found by now, study requires you to do some independent work above and beyond the information provided by your course and resources.

We hope you find the book useful in developing your understanding of the context in which your patients live and the ways in which you can help them live with dignity and autonomy. Good luck with your studies.

Chapter 1 Understanding complex care

Chapter aims

After reading this chapter, you will be able to:

- define complex care and relate it to your own practice
- identify and describe the systemic issues for people living with complexity
- explain the basic benefits that people living with complexity may encounter
- understand the importance of engaging with people living with complexity and, where necessary, their friends and family.

Introduction

'Complex care' is becoming a more frequently used term within healthcare. While the concept of complex care crosses boundaries with long-term conditions (LTC), it requires a different approach. Complex care is often involved when multiple conditions or social circumstances require an approach that is collaborative and based on case management activity. The Department of Health (DH) defines a LTC as: *a condition that cannot, at present, be cured but is controlled by medication and/or other treatment/ therapies* (Department of Health, 2012, p. 4); complex care is focused more broadly on the interactions between the situation the person is in, their health needs and the systems that support them. A person can have one health condition and still have complex needs, since the situation itself can cause the complexity. As a nurse, you will be expected to understand these complexities and be an advocate for your patient, whatever issue is influencing the situation they are living in. You have a duty of care to provide high-quality care and interventions based on their needs and preferences. As you will learn as we travel through this book, this is not always easy.

As the definition and focus of complex care moves from a primarily acute setting to a specialist community one, we find that it becomes less medicalised and more focused on the person and how their situation is impacting their life. Primarily the complexities in this area arise from the overlap between their health condition and their situation, whether that be their ability to navigate health and social care systems or the financial pressures that have arisen from their health. Previously, you might find literature speaking about hip fractures that require a range of healthcare professionals as a complex case. Now, complexity is reflected in the situation of the patient rather than the medical diagnosis. The situations that create complexities and barriers to this coordinated care persist, despite our awareness of the need for care coordination and transitional support.

This chapter will explore the issues around basic definitions, statistics, costs and guidelines. It will discuss the differences in framing complexity from literature to lived experience. Let's explore your initial thoughts about complex care.

Activity 1.1   Critical thinking

Although there is a clear definition of LTC, there may be less common knowledge on the definition of complex care.

When you think of complex care, what are your initial thoughts?

What might a definition include? Create one for yourself before progressing with this chapter.

Thinking of your clinical experience, can you think of patients whose care might be considered complex?

As the answers will be based on your own thoughts, there is no outline answer at the end of this chapter.

As nurses, we have historically worked in teams and, when we decided to write this book, we realised we wanted this to be a team effort. We wanted to make sure the right stories were told and that the most important people were able to influence what we have included. Throughout this book, you will find commentary and stories from our group of experts by experience (EbE). These are people living with long-term or complex conditions who have kindly collaborated on the book with us and will share their thoughts with you as we explore the topics. The NMC now require that the EbE be involved in the training of nursing students.

Box 1.1 Introducing our experts by experience

These people have kindly given up their time to read, comment and collaborate on this book with us. These are their real stories, but in some cases, they have chosen to have a pseudonym.

Rosemary and Harry with Hermione and Eddie

Harry has haemophilia. This is a genetic bleeding disorder and often requires families to become experts in the management of the bleeds. He has a little sister called Hermione and lives with his mother and father. Rosemary, his mother, works part time and his father, Eddie, works full time. They are supported by their families and work with a paediatric specialist team. There is no photograph because it was important to protect Harry and Hermione's identity.

Bettie

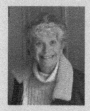

Bettie is a retired cisgendered nurse who trained in Birmingham in the late 1980s. She has clinical experience in ITUs, theatre and general practice and has worked with pharmaceutical companies as a nurse adviser. She retired due to ill health. She is married with two adult children who are both now self-sufficient. She enjoys many hobbies which are arts-based, likes to travel, loves skiing and adores the theatre. She tells us that you can take a girl out of nursing, but you can never take nursing out of a girl!

John

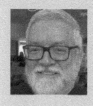

John is a cisgendered man and has multiple long-term conditions that require careful and consistent management. These include hypothyroidism, ischemic heart disease, stage 3 kidney disease, ME/CFS and fibromyalgia. As a result of these energy-limiting conditions he is a powered-wheelchair user.

Colette

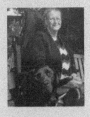 Colette is a cisgendered mother of two grown-up children, grandmother to one girl and widowed after 40 years of marriage. She has a lifelong medical condition called EDS, which stands for Elhors-Danlos spectrum disorder; this is classed as a rare condition and is a fault in the protein gene. Her major problem is her joints which affects her by always having tendonitis – very similar to repetitive strain injury but in all joints (except elbows) all the time with just everyday living. She is double jointed, but her tendons do not tighten up, so she is prone to subluxation or dislocation of her joints and often hypersensitivity around her joints. Cayde is her support animal.

Mark

Mark is an expert by experience with a diagnosis of 'mild learning disabilities'.

Mark has lived his whole life in the South West of England, initially with his parents and then as a young adult in local residential services for people with learning disabilities. In 2013 Mark moved into his own flat near his family and the local church, and has lived there independently ever since. He recieves eight hours per week flexible 1:1 support from an experienced support worker who he employs directly and pays via direct payments. This was a big step in Mark's independence and taking control in his life.

As an expert by experience, Mark works as a visiting lecturer at two universities including the University of Gloucestershire, teaching across a variety of health and social care programmes, and travels independently from his flat in Somerset. Mark has been a long-term advocate for people with learning disabilities and has roles as an ambassador for Positive People Somerset, and Discovery in Somerset. He has recently undertaken a Makaton (sign language) course to be able to better support and advocate for others.

Mark aims to keep up his teaching and his advocacy work for as long as he can, and to make the world a better place for people with learning disabilities.

As well as these true experiences, throughout the book you will find various case studies. These are based around fictional characters we will use to illustrate issues, alongside our experts by experience.

Box 1.2 Complex care at home team

Throughout our book, you will find examples and commentary from a team of healthcare professionals who specialise in complex care, working together to proactively manage the care of people with complex health needs. The services are focused on those who are high users of primary or urgent care services; they use a case-managed approach. A specialist complex care team has kindly contributed to this book, providing case studies and their expertise.

Definitions

On completing activity 1.1, you might have noticed that it was quite hard to define. That is why there are so many definitions from many governments, policies and guidelines. This makes it much harder for this group of patients because they do not sit in a single category that would produce a gold standard for complexity.

The word 'complexity' comes from Latin – complexus – and means how things can be connected and how those things work (or don't) together. The issues that come from those interactions bring with them unpredictability, uncertainty and ambiguity (Lysdahl and Hofmann, 2016).

Several different terms can be found, with overlapping components and uses, making it difficult for us to have a clear picture of who may fall into this group of people. In medical terms, the term focuses on the 'co-morbidity' of diseases as the primary defining feature (Maree et al., 2020). This relies on the medical model being the primary focus of consideration, placing the medical team's perspective of the patient as important, which contradicts the person-centred care approach.

'Multi-morbidity', another term that has a large cross-coverage with complex care, can be either 2+ or 3+ disease entities. This has been overtaken by the use of 'complex multi-morbidity', a term that includes three or more different body systems within one person – a reliable way of identifying patients whose use of healthcare tends to be greater, quality of life is lower and illness is more severe (Harrison et al., 2014). These terms do risk making the disease the centre of our work; it might be better that the terms we use put the person at the centre, which would include a person who has one condition alongside multiple other, complicating factors, such as housing, finances, family dynamics or access to services.

By having a broader viewpoint, including such things as social support, housing and financial situations we can include these concepts, but not centralise them, keeping the person as the primary focus of discussion. This allows us, as clinicians, to consider other issues, which would include the social determinants of health, that are often more important to the patient than a particular long-term condition (Maree et al., 2020).

Manning and Gagnon (2017) explored this concept, demonstrating that a broad variety of terms (Figure 1.1) can be included within complex patients. They refer to these terms as surrogate terms, illustrating the journey from the co-morbidity concept of the 1970s through to the broader, systems-based definition of complex patients, one that considers the person in the context of their conditions, social relationships and environmental factors. In each speciality area different definitions are in use. You will find more information about those specifics in Chapters 8, 9, 10 and 11.

In each of these definitions, there tends to be a focus on the use of healthcare services. Accessing healthcare requires a few factors to be in place. These can be as simple as transport to an outpatient appointment, the ability to interact with the information provided by healthcare staff, or the knowledge of which services are available. Healthcare systems are, by nature, designed around managing acute, single conditions and do not allow for complexity-compatible policy to easily exist (Maree et al., 2020). They do not consider the essential connections with social care and social safety nets that are a vital part of living with complex care needs.

Box 1.3   The Medical Research Council definitions

These focus more on complexity of interventions; dimensions of complexity include:

- *Number of and interactions between components within the experimental and control interventions*
- *Number and difficulty of behaviours required by those delivering or receiving the intervention*
- *Number of groups or organisational levels targeted by the intervention*
- *Number and variability of outcomes*
- *Degree of flexibility or tailoring of the intervention permitted.*

(Medical Research Council, 2019, p. 7)

Overall, no single definition can be found for complex care, but all of these agree that the perspective of the patient must include their situation, the environment and social relationships they have, alongside the medical needs. All these definitions do have a number of things in common. They agree that complex care must be person-centric, speaking of goal setting with an individual and of enabling them to manage their conditions. They recognise that there are structural barriers and that navigation of systems is a barrier. Complex care aims to break through the silo thinking that divides health and social care, medical specialities and locations. It is driven by data, allowing statistics such as hospital admissions to support changes which in turn improve quality of life for patients (National Center for Complex Health and Social Needs, 2017).

For the purposes of this text, we will be using the Grembowski et al. definition: *the misalignment between patient needs and services* (Grembowski et al., 2014, p. 8), but looking at Figure 1.1 may help you visualise some of the factors involved in complex care (Kuipers et al., 2011). This definition allows for people with single healthcare issues who are struggling to get the care they need from the health and social care system and wider services (see Gloria's case study below).

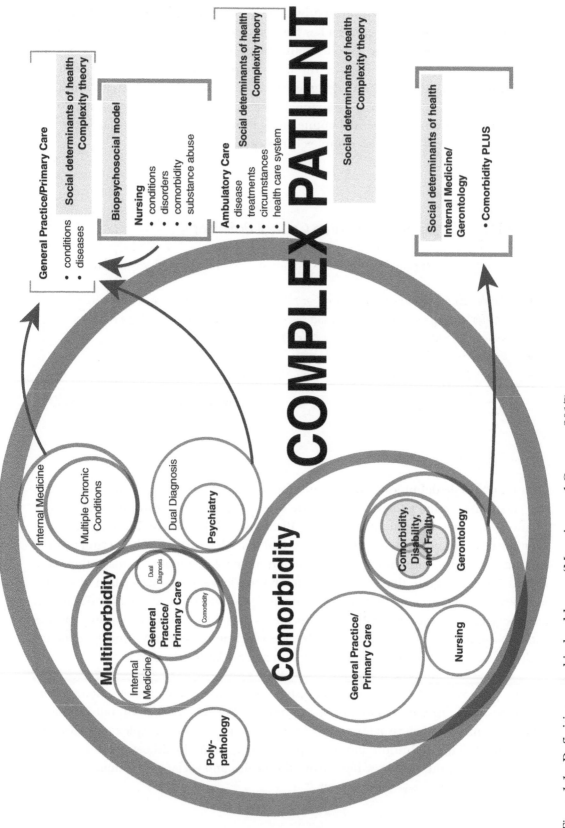

Figure 1.1 Definitions used in healthcare (Manning and Gagnon, 2017)

Case study: Gloria

Gloria is a 36-year-old cisgender woman who is living in temporary housing with her two children. She has had longstanding severe asthma, which has recently worsened. She has had this since she was young and has always self-managed her condition with the support of her practice nurse and GP. She was an ex-smoker but has recently restarted.

Josh is aged ten and Olivia is five. It has been highlighted that the children are missing a considerable number of school days and Olivia has recently developed incontinence.

The housing they have been offered and accepted is a small bed and breakfast with one room and shared amenities. They had to leave their home due to domestic abuse and have very few of their own belongings.

Activity 1.2   Team working

Read the case study above about Gloria and her children and then answer the following questions:

- What about this situation may make the case complex care rather than a single LTC management?
- What impact does Gloria's situation have on her health management?
- Which departments do you think might be involved?

A brief outline answer is given at the end of the chapter.

The Nuffield Trust highlights the lack of coordinated reliable statistics on people living with complexity, particularly in social care. The lack of funding is a primary cause of this reduction in information, as well as the availability of care packages (see Chapter 3). This division of health and social care is exacerbated by the lack of and challenges to collaboration between the two. Poor data prevents quality services from being developed and hinders progress in care. Although some systems are beginning to draw information together, such as the National Social Care Data Portal for Wales, the Nuffield Trust highlights the difficulty in comparing data across systems, given the differences in defining terms such as 'access' – in one system this may mean that the person has been referred and in another it may mean that they have received the care.

Now that complex care is an established field of practice you can find teams in many countries and all of them work across systems to support people living with complexity. It is very difficult to determine precise, realistic and reliable data on the numbers, locations and causes of complexity. This is complicated by the terms used by these teams to classify the patient cohort they treat. For example, in the US you often find terms such as 'complex care management', whereas in Australia it is 'chronic care management'. In the UK, we have no clear guidance for complex care, with many teams focused on admissions to hospitals as the trigger point for entry to their case-load. Throughout this text, we will be using examples and commentary from a team whose design was to counter the barriers created within the system to management of these patients.

Socioeconomic factors impact on multi-morbidity rates: these are significantly higher among deprived populations, particularly those with mental health problems, and the number of conditions influences the use of health services more than the specific diseases (The King's Fund, 2012) (see Chapter 2 for more details).

Healthcare costs

People living with chronic, complex conditions are frequently admitted to hospital, and often readmitted. It is difficult to ascertain how many of the readmissions include people who can be considered complex; there were 865,625 emergency readmissions to hospital within 30 days of discharge in England (figures for 2017–18), many of them involving older people.

It is possible to reduce readmissions with simple interventions, such as contact by a community nursing team (Vernon et al., 2019) (remember our complex care team?). These contacts, followed up as needed with supportive actions such as referrals on to GPs or medication advice, reduced a readmission rate from 15.67 per cent to 9.24 per cent (p = 0.011). A meta-analysis demonstrated the impact of a variety of models that mirror this in reducing emergency admissions, as well as all-cause or condition-specific readmissions (Damery et al., 2016). These interventions included multidisciplinary teams (MDT) that included condition-specific expertise, and the addition of specialist nurses or pharmacists with self-management to the broader interventions. These were more powerful when this happened at someone's home.

There has been a shift, with more care taking place in the community where knowledgeable healthcare professionals can provide guidance, support and education on issues such as self-management, releasing capacity from the acute sector. The growth of experts by experience demonstrates this shift, with the person or their family acting as advocate/s and manager/s of their care, working in partnership with the healthcare team and others (see Chapter 4).

Overall, living with complex health needs brings with it increased costs across all realms of life, from hospital costs, dental care, emergency service use, home adaptation, to primary care appointments (Soley-Bori et al., 2020). We know that those living in more deprived areas have higher risks for poorer health, increased healthcare issues and higher risks of early death. There is an increase of 27 per cent in secondary care costs and 47 per cent in social care costs between affluent and deprived areas (Jayatunga et al., 2019).

Costs can include education, prescriptions, or trips to the hospital, so it is almost impossible to state with any certainty the costs related to complex care. We can extrapolate from other numbers to give us a broad picture of the impact, both to the health services and to the person and their family.

Living with disability

Some organisations have worked to define the costs of living with disability, which can be related to living with complex conditions (Scope, 2019). When we ask people to manage their healthcare, whether that be self-management, attending appointments or buying prescriptions, we expect them to take on the burden of the costs. A fifth of disabled adults had extra costs of more than £1000 a month, even when adjusted for the benefit payments that are intended to meet those costs (Scope, 2019). It is important to consider that the complexity of the person and their situation will impact carers' and families' ability to maintain employment and education. This is the equivalent of a disability tax reducing every £100 of income to £68. This applied to families with disabled children as well; a quarter of them face costs over £1000 a month, average costs of £528 if there is one disabled child, rising to £823 if there are two or more.

The impact of complex conditions on employment can be taken from the impact LTCs in general have in that area (The King's Fund, 2012): people are less likely to be employed, but more so in the latter category. Absences from the workplace have been found to be higher in people with co-morbidities than in people with a single condition and, where the two interact, employment is worsened (The King's Fund, 2012).

Benefits

The welfare state exists to provide practical help and financial support for those who are unemployed and looking for work. It provides people with assistance if their earnings are low, if they have a disability, are bringing up children, are retired, care for someone or are ill. Navigating this complex system is often frustrating and can require knowledge, effort and time. For people with limited amounts of energy, this can be challenging, especially when it changes frequently.

There is a huge variety of different entitlements that may be available to your patient; funding sources are equally complex (see Chapter 3). In children and those with learning disability this is more difficult since a child needs to have already missed milestones; there is delay in identifying this and then applying for funding. This can have a lasting impact on the child and their family, their relationship with their teams and their future well-being. These are some examples of funding streams that your patient may be using, but it is not possible to create a full list as they change frequently, adding to the difficulties of the situation.

Box 1.4 Benefits for complex needs

Continuing healthcare (CHC): a person has been assessed as having a primary health need and it is the NHS's responsibility to provide the assessed healthcare and social needs of the person. An exceptional fund for people with exceptional needs, it is not a mainstream source of NHS funding.

Fast track: when a person has a rapidly declining condition that may be entering end of life, they can then receive CHC without a lengthy assessment process.

Funded nursing care: a payment made by the NHS to a care home for the care provided by a registered nurse.

Specialist placements: when a person has healthcare needs that need specialist care and treatment but is expected to make a degree of recovery.

Joint funding: Clinical commissioning group (CCG), the local authority (LA) or a self-funding person; this is funding when it has been assessed that the NHS ought to contribute towards the cost of care.

Section 117: a provision of aftercare services for certain people who have previously been detained under sections of the Mental Health Act (1983, amended, 2007).

Personal independence payments (PIP): one of the benefits that has come in for a considerable amount of criticism, with frequent statistics released showing that 76 per cent of appeals are successful (more in Chapter 3).

Activity 1.3   Critical thinking

Read the case study about Gloria and then answer the following:

- What benefits might she be entitled to?
- What costs might she incur compared to people who are not living with a disability?

A brief outline answer is given at the end of the chapter.

In the following case studies, you might gain some insight into the impact of finances on those living with complexity or their parents or carers.

Case study: Simeon

Simeon, a 47-year-old, transgender man, has primary progressive multiple sclerosis; he is now struggling to manage his care and has poor mobility. Previously he had received both aspects of PIP at a high level. This year, his application was denied for the mobility aspect. The impact of having to go to appeal was stressful, affecting his health; he was unable to ask his family to help him with his finances while he waited for the appeal (which would have been very helpful), so his appeal had an instant impact. His case was reviewed and his application was approved.

As well as formal, visible costs, such as purchasing equipment or paying bills, families may incur other hidden costs. There may be impacts of the unpredictability of conditions which can cause major financial problems for them.

Case study: Harry

As a child with haemophilia, Harry may have bleeds unexpectedly. It is expected that he will need treatment for occasions such as a tooth extraction but, as a child, he may injure himself during play or as he lives his life. It has been important to Rosemary and her family that he is not wrapped in cotton wool to protect him but allowed to exist as a child. Should Harry fall over and bang his head at school (as many school children do!), he would have to go to a children's hospital where they are familiar with haemophilia for a check and potentially for treatment.

Activity 1.4   Critical thinking

In the case study above, Rosemary may be required to leave work abruptly to take her child to the hospital, without warning or ability to plan. Consider what impacts this might have on the financial situation for this family.

A brief outline answer is given at the end of the chapter.

Guidelines

There is no one NICE guideline regarding complex care, but more specific pathways are available for monitoring a condition and managing the symptoms with the aim of improving the quality of life for the patient. The complexity of care can arise from a single condition or with the presence of multiple conditions interacting; the NICE multi-morbidity guideline considers optimising the care for adults with multi-morbidity which can be complex by reducing treatment burden and unplanned care. These guidelines highlight the value of shared decision-making with the emphasis on what is important in terms of treatment, health priorities, lifestyle and goals.

Guidelines set the standard to provide the best care for the patient, as well as identifying gaps and areas of improvement nationally. The NICE guideline 'Transition from Children's to Adult Services' has resulted in a requirement to plan how a young adult patient transitions, allowing the young person involvement in the decisions and the adjustments to changes to their future care. Early transition planning is now supported by legal requirements and is covered by health, social care and education legislation (see Chapter 10).

There have been several pilots that consider a tailored approach to the treatment of an individual who has a complex care need. In 2014, the 'Health 1000' pilot established a dedicated multidisciplinary team of NHS healthcare and voluntary sector professionals that were recruited into the practice, including GPs, nurses, physiotherapists, occupational therapists, pharmacists and social workers. In Gloucestershire, the complex care team works in a very similar way, drawing together health and social care into a multidisciplinary team. You can read more about the way this works in Chapter 6.

Activity 1.5   Evidence-based practice and research

Since there is no guideline related to complex care management, what might you include within one, should you oversee writing one?

A brief outline answer is given at the end of the chapter.

Nurses will care for patients in a range of situations. We look after them in the acute sector, where they may be receiving care for their condition, or for another unrelated issue. They may be in adult or child acute services. They may be in the community, where nurses may engage with them in GP practices, specialist community-based teams, or in community nursing.

In child services there has been a move towards family-centred care, as part of the general focus on person-centred care (see more about this in Chapter 10). The family dynamics can be part of the complexity, throughout people's lives, but for families with children this is more central. There is a large transfer of care to the parents, making them responsible for their child's care needs; we can, as healthcare professionals, only react to the picture before us, at the time we engage with them (see Chapter 10). Often, we cannot predict disease trajectories and in child health cannot identify the issues until milestones are missed, compared to adults who develop a condition later in life, where we see deterioration.

Increased caregiving is strongly linked to the adverse psychosocial impacts, and family-centred support seeks to hold and support the family throughout their circumstances (Woodgate et al., 2015). The need to be seen as 'good' can impact on the family in many ways, including the presentation at clinic – many of our patients come to clinic in their Sunday best, presenting a different situation than the home picture.

In fact, although some literature suggests that time spent on managing conditions can range from 30 minutes a day to two hours (Yen et al., 2013), other studies note that time spent on self-care is directly linked to income (Forbes et al., 2016). This can be transferred to living with a complex condition, since, when you think about it, with increased income you have increased ability to use the assistance of paid services. Without that income you might spend considerable amounts of time, money and energy managing your health.

Case study: complex care team

In many locations in the UK you can find complex care teams. Their aim is to help people avoid hospital and they do this by providing a variety of both clinical and social input 'year of care' approach (care planning) (more on this in Chapter 4).

In Gloucestershire, they have integrated community teams (ICTs) who bring together community nurses, occupational therapists, physiotherapists, social workers and reablement workers to work as one team to serve a local area. These teams work alongside GPs to provide care for people in their place of residence or in the community. They work with the ward teams based in the community hospitals across Gloucestershire and with the countywide specialist services, voluntary organisations and other care providers to provide assessments, treatment and support for people within the community.

In Greater Manchester, the complex care team is based in a primary care network (a group of GPs serving a population of 30,000–50,000 people) and comprises of complex care nurses, care coordinations, pharmacists, adult, child and adolescent mental health nurses, paramedics, social prescribers and a cancer care and early diagnosis nurse. As with the Gloucestershire team, they work alongside the GP,

These are just two examples of this type of team. There are many others within the NHS; more in Chapter 5.

Activity 1.6   Reflection

After reading this initial chapter, return to your first reflection. How has the new information changed your views on complex care? Did you consider the broader context when you first reflected?

As this activity is based on your own reflection, there is no outline answer at the end of this chapter.

Within complex care, the people are varied in condition, situation and demographic, from children to adults, from mental to physical health, and those whose lives are impacted by situations that have become medicalised. For all these people, wherever they are, they must navigate complicated healthcare systems that do not come with a manual or map. They must understand the key terms used within and an expert guide who can support them in meeting the needs they themselves set is vital. This need is often met in specialist care coordination teams, with a variety of names. Like those found in LTC care, these can have a massive impact of reducing healthcare costs (to both the patient and the system) and improving quality of life.

Activity 1.7   Decision-making

Thinking about your current or most recent placement, what do you think might trigger a referral to a team that can do a complex care management?

As the answers will be based on your own thoughts, there is no outline answer at the end of this chapter.

Chapter summary

In this chapter, we have looked at the broad topic of complex care and what it is. We have introduced some people you will find throughout the book and who have kindly given us their knowledge, experience and wisdom as we wrote this book. In the next chapter, we'll look at the context of complex care, exploring social and political determinants of health.

Activities: brief outline answers

Activity 1.2 Team working (page 11)

The social and living situation for Gloria and her children are the factors that make this a complex case. The socioeconomics are impacting her health and this is creating a spiral which cannot be improved without multidisciplinary working.

The stress has caused her to return to smoking, using a coping mechanism to manage, and the habitat is worsening her asthma, with the potential of triggers in the house itself such as mould or allergies. This, combined with the stress of their situation and the abrupt house move – with associated emotional loss and grief – is impacting on the whole family.

Care could involve:

- the school
- GP and practice nurse
- health visitor
- social services, including child services and a case worker for domestic violence
- voluntary services such as domestic violence support network or patient groups.

Activity 1.3 Critical thinking (page 14)

Read the case study above about Gloria and her family and then consider the following:

- she would receive Universal Credit (possibly around £194 per week, with a five-week wait at the time of writing);
- she would receive some housing benefit but there is a cap called the Local Housing Allowance rate;
- she would be entitled to Child Benefit;
- she may receive Council Tax support;
- she may get Disability Living Allowance or Scottish Child Disability Payment.

It is worth noting that they may have left their home with little, and may have no reserves to pay for private housing deposit or new furniture, clothes, etc.

Activity 1.4 Critical thinking (page 15)

With unexpected treatment, his parents must find work that is flexible to allow them to leave work abruptly. There are also hidden costs such as fuel and parking, and some treatment supplies are not covered by the NHS. There may be unexpected childcare costs for those without family or friends able to pick up his sister at short notice.

Activity 1.5 Critical thinking (page 16)

You would consider issues such as the MDT and the ability of the patient to access them swiftly at the point of need – self-referral might be useful here. You might also consider having benefit advisers and care coordinators as a standard part of the primary care team.

Annotated further reading

Kuluski, K., Ho, J. W., Hans, P. K. and Nelson, M. L. (2017). Community care for people with complex care needs: bridging the gap between health and social care. *International Journal of Integrated Care*, 17(4). https://doi.org/10.5334/ijic.2944

Read this article for insights into the gap between health and social care.

Useful websites

https://www.kingsfund.org.uk/projects/co-ordinated-care-people-complex-chronic-conditions

Read about the projects that have taken place to work with care coordination for people with complex chronic conditions.

https://www.kingsfund.org.uk/publications/co-ordinated-care-people-complex-chronic-conditions

This website discusses the types of service engaged with people living with complex needs and which indicators are important.

Chapter 2   Complex care in context

Chapter aims

After reading this chapter, you will be able to:

- identify some of the social, political and broader issues that impact on people living with complex conditions
- consider the biological and psychological drivers
- identify the policies and procedures that exist
- understand the mitigating factors that nursing can provide to support those people.

Introduction

We have talked about the definitions of complex care, and costs of living with complex needs. Now we will be exploring the social and political context, examining the biological and psychological drivers behind complex needs, and looking at some of the factors in nursing that might have an impact, such as polypharmacy, policies and procedures. Cajal sums up the issues we will discuss: *Every disease has two causes. The first is pathophysiological; the second, political* (Brant, 1993, p. 12).

We should explore the other forces such as social, economic, healthcare, behavioural, genetic and environmental, without going further, drawing back and looking at the whole systems (Dawes, 2020). Since complex conditions are those where the system does not match the needs of the person, this is a vital part of understanding the drivers behind those issues.

Given this need to look at the broader context, it is important that we understand the sociology of health, since the time spent with the health services makes up a tiny amount of a person's life compared to the time that they spend living with complex needs. We will look at the impacts of these broader powers in society and how they might act on our patients' lives. As we do this, we will explore the experience of Howard.

Case study: Howard

Howard, an 84-year-old cisgender man, was being regularly admitted to hospital with frequent falls and issues around caring for his needs at home. He had several services involved but was referred to the complex care team to treat him more holistically.

When they visited, they identified several key issues and interventions for Howard: he was found to be experiencing long-term depression and was very socially isolated. It took a few visits for him to admit that he needed some help and accept the services and interventions that were offered.

He lived in a first-floor flat and struggled to get up the stairs. He did not have facilities to wash his clothes, or items that would allow him to clean his flat effectively.

He lived alone, having lost his partner some time ago. He admitted he was very lonely.

Drivers in complex care

A driver is something that acts as a catalyst for change in society. That might be as simple as a governmental policy deciding what type of personal protective equipment to wear or a change in the NMC guidelines. It might be about the person themselves, whether that be psychological or physical. In this chapter, we will explore a few different types of drivers that act in complex care.

Sociological drivers

Sociology is the interaction between individuals, social environments and society (Barry and Yuill, 2016). Those factors influence our beliefs and our behaviours, teaching us how our society and culture think it is appropriate to respond to a situation. You will have heard of several models in the way we work in health – the medical model or the social model are examples of this. The medical model focuses on disease, the pathophysiology and the specific biological cause. It considers changes from 'the normal', including the signs and symptoms, and focuses on the presentation of those to the medical team (Gabe and Monaghan, 2013). The social model takes a different approach; it focuses on the attitudes and structures of society that disable people with medical conditions, so it aligns well with the Equality Act (2010). The biopsychosocial model was originally created by Engel, but changes have been made since then, since criticisms suggested it was too vague and lacking in a scientific basis (Bolton and Gillett, 2019). Evidence has come to support it; social determinants of health demonstrating the link between the social, adverse childhood experiences showing that childhood experiences impact on health, and lifestyles becoming more strongly linked as risks or protective factors in health (Bolton and Gillett, 2019).

In addition, the intersection of these things can worsen the harm caused; for example, race and gender intersects for women of colour and means that the social and cultural capital they have is less than either white women or men of colour. Race increases or decreases the likelihood of being diagnosed with severe mental illnesses and this has often been presented as a fact caused by individual choices, rather than systemic and interpersonal racism (Nazroo et al., 2020). The inequalities throughout the world on every level – social, economic and political – bring with them negative health outcomes. There are differences in the treatment people receive, with increased compulsory admission and police involvement in health for people who are black; work by Nazroo et al. (2020) makes it clear that 'othering' and inequalities are a direct result of the structural issues in our society. As an example of that, the primary barrier to safe healthcare (such as hormonal therapy) for transgender people is the lack of providers with expertise in that area (Safer et al., 2016). This group faces multiple health disparities and stigma, and waiting eighteen months for the first appointment at a specialist centre adds to that burden.

You might think about the Bristol Social Exclusion Matrix here (do a quick search for this work by academics at Bristol University), which shows the impact of resources on our ability to participate and our quality of life. Social exclusion is about the person's ability to be part of the social, economic, political, or cultural life, and therefore their ability to relate to others. You can explore the matrix across the four stages of life: childhood, youth, working-age adult and later life. The three domains on the matrix are areas of potential importance which may impact on a person's life. Where a person has a high level of resources, they can participate in life and their quality of life subsequently improves, and the opposite is true.

Again, intersectionality applies here – over the course of a life, this discrimination accumulates. The earlier the discrimination, the greater the impact across the lifespan (Holman and Walker, 2020). Holman and Walker go on to note that policy contexts including austerity, neoliberalism and commercial interests directly relate to the inequalities. But an example can be found in higher education – the disparity between those of an advantaged background compared to a disadvantaged one is striking there. You could consider the use of food banks, access to motorised disability vehicles, or the ability to live safely during a pandemic (use of food delivery, access to working from home, etc.). The latter suggests that poverty and social exclusion is relative, a sliding scale. Townsend (cited in Towsend et al., 2020) describes the subjectivity as someone lacking the resources to engage in the type of activities that are customary in the society that they live in. His deprivation indicators ranged from lacking meals on a day in the last fortnight to not having a fridge. Given that was in 1968, we have not moved so far from those needs being lacking in our society! We know that, from the Marmot report, only one third of health is caused by traditional, biological risk factors; the rest is caused by society (Marmot, 2020).

Activity 2.1   Reflection

Consider Marmot's statistic around choice. What other determinants of health might prevent people from making choices? Can you link them to the Bristol Social Exclusion Matrix?

Although this activity is based on your own thoughts, a brief outline answer is provided at the end of this chapter.

So, the importance of the model we select matters: while the medical model focuses on that third of factors, the social model puts the health of the person into a social context. The biopsychosocial model considers the factors such as poor housing, life experiences and other triggers that, alongside biological systems, create issues for people. It becomes clearer that inequality makes society less cohesive, less functional, less democratic, less successful economically and less healthy. Marmot published an article in a newspaper (2022) pointing out that the cuts to those on benefits during this year and inflation impact a person on every level, but that changes such as affordability of housing, transport and food improve society and health (Marmot, 2022).

Activity 2.2   Critical thinking

Revisit the story of Howard and consider which social determinants of health are impacting on his life.

Although this activity is based on your own thoughts, a brief outline answer is provided at the end of this chapter.

Political drivers

Since inequality is a major driver, the political determinants of health are equally as important as social determinants; the two are linked so strongly that it is difficult to separate them. The political determinants focus on the system, relationships, resources and power interactions and processes. The model that Dawes identified examined the ways those drivers interact, considering voting, government and policy. These issues are not new, with literature going back to 2001 where researchers have tried to move that focus from the person or the biology behind the issues to draw attention to the impact of governmental policy (Mackenbach, 2014). If we do not examine the political determinants, we ignore an important factor in the social determinants of health and the inequalities that are related to both – we have combined them into one model to show the interconnectivity (Figure 2.1). Despite this, Mackenbach (2014) sounded a note of caution: good evidence requires controls, and that is very difficult in country-level, policy-driven, politically related health. You cannot easily divide a country in two and provide good social housing in one and not the other without people simply moving into the better location.

There is no simple direct link between increased expenditure and improvement in health of a society. The clear link to politics is shown in our adapted framework of the political determinants of health. Dawes' framework lists several political determinants of health, which interplay to impact on the health of those living in the country. Therefore, political ideology, which identifies societal problems and how to manage them, decides the timing and manner of not only the policy but also how it is formed (Bryant, 2013).

Many nursing researchers have focused on the political determinants of health, examining how government actions and policy relate to inequality and health outcomes, either directly or indirectly. When we speak of people being vulnerable, the image of risk, harm or fragility comes to mind – this ignores the systemic inequalities that create the situation the person is in (Aday, 2001, cited by Dickman and Chicas, 2021). Dickman and Chicas (2021) speak about this, highlighting that the rhetoric around 'vulnerable' populations included nurses themselves, spoken of as heroes and angels in the Covid-19 pandemic, which made us appear as those giving up their lives willingly, as sacrifice. Terms such as vulnerable population can undermine the power of that group, removing their autonomy, making them more likely to receive condescension and paternalism, side-lining them from political power. Nurses are well positioned to advocate for the changes our patients need, to correct the inequalities within our systems. Dickman and Chicas (2021) note that work should be as a partnership rather than including them as interesting subjects to be studied. But social and political determinants include a complex landscape of other drivers, such as the biological and psychological.

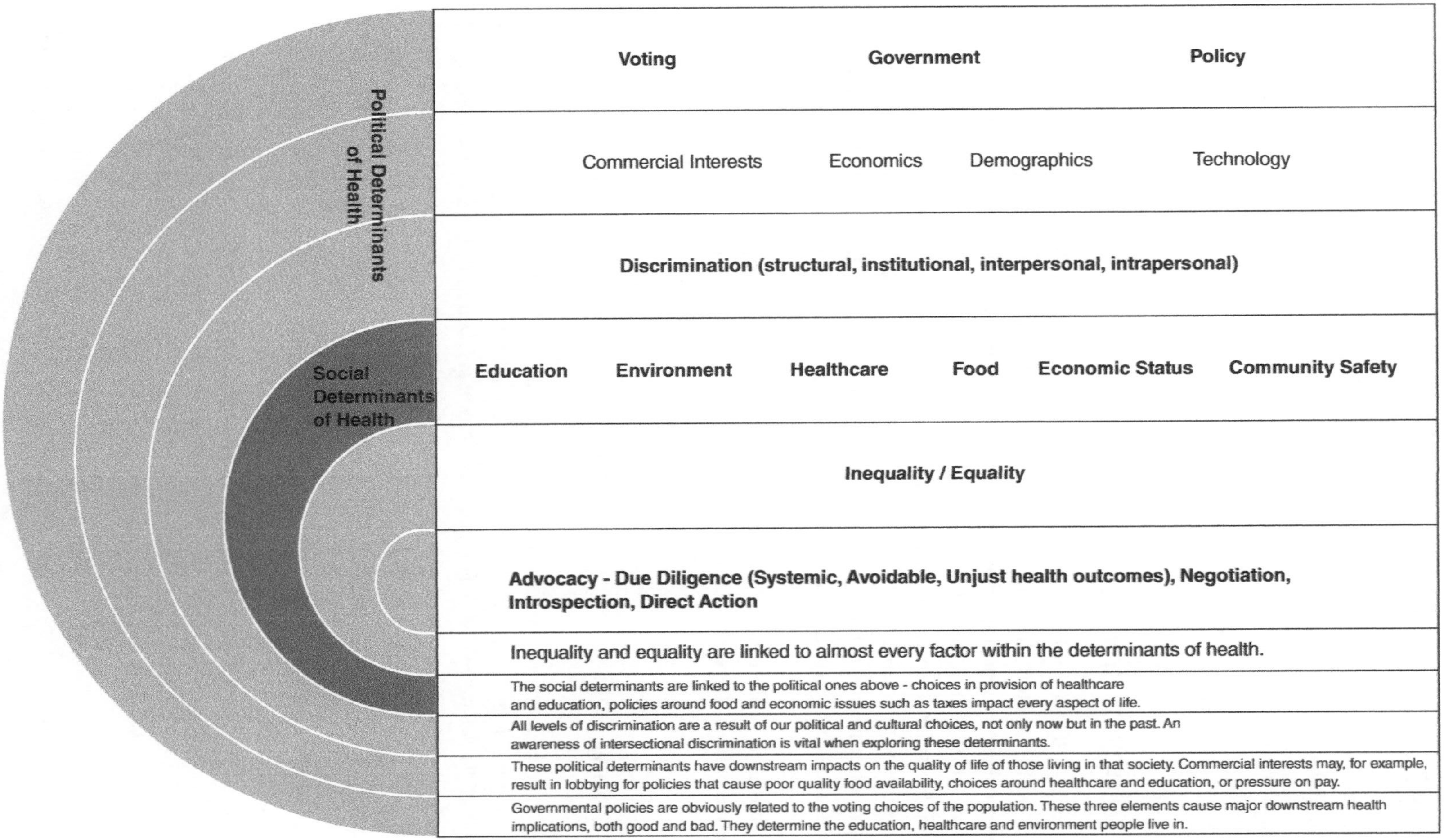

Voting

Government

Policy

Commercial Interests   Economics   Demographics   Technology

Discrimination (structural, institutional, interpersonal, intrapersonal)

Education   Environment   Healthcare   Food   Economic Status   Community Safety

Inequality / Equality

Advocacy - Due Diligence (Systemic, Avoidable, Unjust health outcomes), Negotiation, Introspection, Direct Action

Inequality and equality are linked to almost every factor within the determinants of health.

The social determinants are linked to the political ones above - choices in provision of healthcare and education, policies around food and economic issues such as taxes impact every aspect of life.

All levels of discrimination are a result of our political and cultural choices, not only now but in the past. An awareness of intersectional discrimination is vital when exploring these determinants.

These political determinants have downstream impacts on the quality of life of those living in that society. Commercial interests may, for example, result in lobbying for policies that cause poor quality food availability, choices around healthcare and education, or pressure on pay.

Governmental policies are obviously related to the voting choices of the population. These three elements cause major downstream health implications, both good and bad. They determine the education, healthcare and environment people live in.

Political Determinants of Health

Social Determinants of Health

Figure 2.1   Political and social determinants of health (adapted from Dawes, 2020; Marmot, 2014)

Activity 2.3 Critical thinking

Revisit the story of Howard and consider which political determinants of health are impacting on his life.

Although this activity is based on your own thoughts, a brief outline answer is provided at the end of this chapter.

Psychological drivers

Cheng et al. (2019) spoke about the psychological need for people to exist in a certain role within society, linking the need to be able to be productive, whether that be in housework or in working. Equally, having relationships is a key psychological driver; in our previous scenario of Howard, we explored the experience of a man who was very socially isolated and the impact that contact and activity had on his well-being. Relationships with friends and family are important, but also it is important for people living with complexity to have a good relationship with their health professionals. Being able to discuss their situation and weigh up the difficult choices as part of a team is key. Feeling respected and comfortable with their team makes it possible to have those vital conversations; it took time for Howard to allow his team to help him. Consider Bettie's experience below, where she felt disrespected and deceived by her team.

Case study: Bettie

After years of being treated by the community mental health team (CMHT) and having been labelled with various different diagnoses, a consultant psychiatrist decided that he was going to prescribe me Clozapine. I researched the medication and decided that I didn't want to take it as I felt it would not help me. His response at the appointment when I told him this was 'Are you sure you're even ill, then, if you won't take the tablets?' At this same appointment, I mentioned in conversation that I thought my children, aged seventeen and fourteen, hated me. I later found out that the team had contacted social services and reported me as a concern to them. They hadn't contacted my GP, nor my husband, nor even the children's schools. At no point did I feel part of a team. I felt as if I was being dictated to. As the victim of years of childhood sexual abuse, I was treated as if I was the problem rather than being treated as a woman with problems. I was judged, blamed and felt regarded as the criminal instead of the victim of the criminal. To compound my distrust, my medical notes were faxed to an electrical store in my local town. The CMHT had given the GP the wrong fax number. An apology was sent to the GP practice and to the electrical store but not to me, the patient. How could I trust these people?

This type of treatment led me to removing myself from the system and finding help from a charity instead – a charity that allowed me to feel part of that team and respected me. Most importantly, I trusted them.

Families are a key element in living with complexity. Whether they are supportive and helpful, or a source of conflict, they have an impact. The family's ability to understand the requirements and impact of the complex needs can be a major factor in the person's life (see chapters 7, 8, 9, and 10).

The person's own perception of their situation and illness matters as well; psychologically, their perceptions may not match up with that of others, including their team and their family. Something that appears small to others may feel insurmountable to the person living with it and vice versa. Their own emotions can impact on their coping processes; they may feel sad, anxious, or depressed but positive in using other skills such as prayer, distraction or humour. Information is vital to them and the healthcare team should be mindful of that need, considering with the person how much they want to receive and the format it should be delivered in (Cheng et al., 2019). This is vital in complex conditions since the information and priorities change over time as the person's situation and needs change.

When we consider this in the different groups we can see how this might have an impact. A child growing up has different needs at four to fifteen. Someone living with mental health issues may find that their needs are different at times. Someone with learning disabilities may change in their needs as their skills change. In each case, decision-making and information needs have changed over time. Psychological needs have evolved and therefore our behaviour should change to meet that.

In some areas, such as mental health, the psychological factors are the cause of the complexity. This is not only the case in mental health conditions but also in areas where stigmatising behaviour may become an issue. Perception by our society of certain conditions as more dangerous, or attracting more prejudice than others, means that this often happens. In all fields, certain conditions are 'blamed', such as HIV, hepatitis C, emotionally unstable personality disorder, or behaviours perceived as attention seeking, which may even find stigma within the healthcare team.

Biological drivers

Complex care can be driven by a mismatch in treatments or needs for two or more conditions; this is known as co-morbidity or multi-morbidity. People are not only living longer but also conditions that were once untreatable are now chronic in nature. A third of patients admitted to hospitals as emergencies have five or more conditions, when this was once only the case for a tenth of admissions; this drives policy for the integrated care systems proposed by the Health and Care White Paper (Department of Health and Social Care, 2021b), which we will explore later in the chapter.

Complexity can be driven by the conditions themselves. Mental and physical health affect each other; those with mental health illnesses have increased risks of obesity, diabetes and cardiovascular disease. Depression worsens diabetes outcomes, both because of the potential for medication concordance to be low and directly on glucose levels

(National Institute for Health Research, 2021). Antiretroviral therapies for HIV and psychotropic drugs are linked to changes within the body that increase the risk of diabetes and cardiovascular diseases.

This increase in co-morbidities is reflected in other countries as well (25 per cent in the US, 37 per cent in Australia) and it is clear from the research and from the personal narratives that living with multiple chronic conditions reduces quality of life and increases costs. Sells et al. (2009, cited in Cheng et al., 2019) stated that living with multiple chronic conditions is a 'virtual cascade of medical, emotional and social hardships' (Cheng et al., 2019, p. 2). Although this speaks to chronic, long-term conditions, it equally applies to people with complex needs since they exist within the same systems. They must attempt to maintain a 'normal' life for themselves, manage their attitudes, balance their medications and cope in a society that is not designed for their needs. Although Cheng et al.'s work is based in the US where the pressures of healthcare costs exist, the same difficulties do arise for people in the UK.

Medication in complexity

When you explore the biological and psychological drivers in health, you begin to look at the individual and how those drivers affect their lives. In any health condition, you are likely to find drivers that relate to medication. Those drivers can be evidence-based, policy-based or polemically based. Consider policies around prescribing; whether they are related to concordance (agreement on what medication to take, when to take it and how much), polypharmacy (many different medications being taken which may interact), or side-effects of the medication (they impact the person at the centre of the work).

When medication is prescribed, it relies on their agreement and ability to take it as prescribed; this agreement between the person and the prescriber is known as concordance or compliance. We prefer to avoid the last word since it implies that the person is doing as they are told and there is strong evidence that people who are engaged and involved in the decision-making process for their healthcare are more likely to take the medication as prescribed (Ng et al., 2018). It is therefore important that communication and trust occur in the appointments where the course of action is agreed – a strong therapeutic alliance is key. Patients who have felt involved will often have more positive attitudes towards taking the medication and feel that they have made an informed choice in their own care. This informed decision should include the risks related to the medication itself. You can see from John's comments (Activity 2.4) and Bettie's story (the second scenario in this chapter) that it is easy for medication changes to be a risk to the health and well-being of the person themselves if we do not take a holistic view of them. But simple moments can prevent other medication errors from occurring, as you will be able to see in the case of John.

Case study: John

I was prescribed a medication to treat depression that would have interacted with the beta and calcium channel blockers I take for my heart condition with potentially fatal results! Thankfully, this was spotted by my pharmacist and the medication was changed.

Activity 2.4   Reflection

In John's case (above), a patient was prescribed the incorrect medication, but a major issue was prevented. Simple actions by the healthcare team matter a good deal.

Reflect for a moment on the cases you see in practice and where the healthcare system may miss the potential interactions in medications and disease.

As this activity is based on your own reflection, no outline answer is given at the end of this chapter.

Many medications, when used over a long time, have an impact on the physical health of the person, sometimes causing further harm to biological systems: long-term use of antipsychotics increases the risks of diabetes and cardiac problems (Correll et al., 2015) and the antiretroviral therapies for HIV are linked to increased insulin resistance, elevated blood lipids and central fat accumulation (Thienemann et al., 2013). So, even in isolation, the medications can be causing harm to those taking them. If you then add another, and another, you have polypharmacy (Masnoon et al., 2017). This has, like many other things in health, many definitions but a generally accepted one is five or more medications daily; there is a balance between appropriate and inappropriate polypharmacy. You might find that some medications were prescribed for side-effects of medications that have been stopped – but the former continue due to the lack of a review. But you may find that some are essential to the well-being of the person taking them and removing them would cause issues that impact on their daily lives.

A medication review and rationalisation are important parts of care, and the person must be included. There are times where a person might resist having medication changes; there are often good reasons for this. Imagine if your well-being and ability to function relied on medications and someone suggests changing one of them. Even a simple change such as the appearance of the medication can have an impact on whether the person takes their medication or not (Lumbreras and López-Pintor, 2017). For people with complex care needs, they are often managing their conditions and situations on several fronts – a change in medication could feel like a risk to them, destabilising a situation that is delicately balanced. It equally could be a welcome relief from symptoms or side-effects that were worsening their situation. Working collaboratively when reviewing medications is a vital part of the nursing role.

Case study: John

I was taking three tablets in this category for several years before the surgery pharmacist did a thorough review and spotted that I was taking them unnecessarily. It reduced the size of my polyphar-macy significantly!

Reviewing medications does include whether people are taking them; self-reported concordance is difficult, since we know that many people do not take their medication as prescribed (Monnette et al., 2018). Be mindful that this is not often deliberate but may stem from the competing demands on their energy when balancing the workload of living with complex needs. That lack of concordance can have many impacts, including worsening of their condition, treatments not working, additional hospital admissions and death (Monnette et al., 2018).

Measurement of that concordance can be completed in a few ways. The frequency of prescription requests from the GP gives a clear indication if the person is taking more than prescribed but does not inform us if the person has not cancelled the repeat that arrives at their home every month or so. Self-reported concordance is often inaccurate, for various reasons, including fear of the consequences. Electronic monitoring devices are one option but are expensive and often just agree with the person's responses.

In older person medicine, there are protocols and guidelines built around the STOPP-START toolkit: that is the 'Screening Tool of Older People's potentially inappropriate Prescriptions' and 'Screening Tool to Alert doctors to Right i.e., appropriate, indicated Treatments' (O'Mahony et al., 2014). Go to Activity 2.5 and consider this tool in terms of your own practice and patients you have worked with.

Activity 2.5   Evidence-based practice

STOPP-START

Look the above toolkit up. In your current or last placement, are/were any of these medications familiar to you?

Consider where you might use this in practice. Challenging medication as a student nurse may be difficult but you can form your thoughts in the shape of a question.

As this activity is based on your own thoughts, no outline answer is given at the end of this chapter.

As we mentioned at the beginning of this section, improvements and changes in this area of practice can often come from policy and procedures that reflect the political and evidence-based care of the day. The resulting policy and procedure of any government has an impact in health – in last decade alone, the laws and policy initiatives found in Box 2.1 have been launched.

Box 2.1   Law and policy initiatives

- Race Relations Amendment Act 2000
- Equality Act 2010
- NHS Equality Delivery System, revised in 2013
- Workforce Race Equality Standard, 2015
- Public Health Outcomes Framework 2010
- Outcome Framework Equity Reports
- NHS Constitution
- Care Quality Commission Standards and Inspection Framework
- Equally Outstanding – Care Quality Commission
- Our Human Rights Approach for Our Health Inequalities – Care Quality Commission
- Assurance Operating Manual for Clinical Commissioning Groups
- Regulation of Health and Social Care Services

(Chouhan and Nazroo, 2020)

These laws and drivers, such as the Marmot report which highlighted the inequalities in health, resulted in a flurry of policies and procedures. Despite these, the inequalities are as apparent in 2020 as they were in 2010 when his report was published (Chouhan and Nazroo, 2020).

Events are another of the driving factors in policy development. In the UK, events such as the Mid Staffordshire NHS Foundation Trust Public Enquiry (2013), otherwise known as the Francis Report, have been key in influencing changes in healthcare. The national strategy for nursing (NHS England, 2014) pointed to the Francis Report (2013), the Keogh Report (2013) and the Berwick Review (2013) as reasons for the NHS to refocus on the core values, putting compassion at the centre again (NHS England, 2014). The Confidential Inquiry into premature deaths of people with learning disabilities (2013) and cases such as Oliver McGowan are examples of such drivers within learning disabilities. These events demonstrated that deaths in people living with a learning disability were often earlier, and the lack of reasonable adjustments was a common factor in this (Heslop et al., 2013). Another report, *Healthcare for All*, recommended that all healthcare professionals should receive training in caring for people with a learning disability (Michael, 2008). Oliver's Campaign also worked towards that goal, and was central to creating the education package that has been rolled out throughout the NHS (Oliver's Campaign, n.d.).

Maintaining Momentum (Parliamentary and Health Service Ombudsman, 2018) demonstrated that, despite policies such as the Five Year Forward View, mistakes in the care of patients have a devastating impact on them, including death. This is often related to their physical healthcare needs not being fully explored or treated. NHS England provided a clear mandate to give parity between physical and mental healthcare, bringing both into a single integrated care system (The King's Fund, 2015). The King's Fund identified the gap between the policies and the reality in the services for people with mental health issues, who are 23 per cent of the burden of disease, but only 11 per cent of the health budget.

Theis and White (2021) found, after reviewing government strategies (1992–2020) that the resulting policies were proposed in ways that prevented their implementation – relying on people to change their behaviours, rather than changing the external factors. If we revisit the social and political determinants of health, many of those factors cannot be influenced by individuals, so this habit of suggesting policies that are little different to the ones that came before suggests the issues are a result of the design, creating barriers to implementation and evaluation. This may explain why determinants of health are not addressed (Byrne et al., 2020); looking at inequality as single issues, rather than multiple connected issues, including the full structural and societal factors that drive them, reduces the chances of actual change. Despite this, changes in politics and policies have a large impact on the factors which influence care; let us take the place of care as an example.

The social policy changed to become 'care in the community' for groups of people living in long-term care, moving those people from institutions – some of which were homes in which those people were settled – into community housing. This idea has been around a long time but in the 1980s the Thatcher government put it into action, using the Griffiths Report to fix the grey area of continuing care of groups that were unable to care for themselves, such as older people, disabled people, or those with long-term mental illness. The following White Paper promoted the independent sector, defined the roles of agencies and pushed towards domiciliary, day and respite care instead of institutions. Changes in the way we talk about these homes or the philosophy of care do not change the circumstances of the patient – sometimes it is simply a change in dwelling, unless there is an actual community for the person to move into. The resulting 'needs assessments' were strongly criticised as interpreting the needs of the person to fit the resources the local government had available to them. Control of personal budgets, where the person has control of their funding, was designed to change that (NHS England, 2019b).

The House of Care (more later on this) is another policy driver that is still working towards changing commissioning for people living with long-term and complex conditions; this speaks of ensuring the person is at the centre, that the care provided suits their needs rather than providing the same menu of care for all (Coulter et al., 2013). It does not include social care within that umbrella, and more recent developments such as the sustainability and transformation plans (STPs) and integrated care systems (ICS) began the move to include both health and social care under the same system (we'll revisit the House of Care model in more detail when we reach Chapter 4).

STPs were policies directed by NHS England in 2015, examining and changing NHS spending and the way it worked with social care and local authorities. The focus was population health and well-being, quality of services and healthcare efficiency (Alderwick et al., 2016). There was some concern at the time that the focus may well be on the latter, with risks to the first two. Alderwick et al. (2016) recognised that the context meant that organisation of care was fragmented, and that working together was increasingly difficult with limited resources. This fragmentation was a direct result of the Health and Social Care Act. It was very clear that NHS staff were experiencing change fatigue with a history of short-term policies.

Despite the concerns, ICS trialled from 2018 in fourteen areas across the country. In general, integrated care models require case managers and routine information-sharing. Case managers are not uncommon in the UK (78 per cent of GP practices (The King's Fund, 2014)) but information-sharing is a frequent issue (7 per cent of GPs stating that other providers did not share information and only 38 per cent shared electronic records).

Activity 2.6   Team working

Consider Howard's case at the start of the chapter and then answer the following:

- What about this situation may make the case complex care rather than a single LTC management?
- What interventions might help Howard?
- Which members of the complex care team do you think might be involved?
- Who might they need to share information with?

A brief outline answer is given at the end of the chapter.

The concept of the complex care team was one of these trials, with a design for the NHS and the social care providers to work closely together. Reviews of ICS demonstrated reduced hospital use, when the organisations involved care navigation, acute home visiting services and intensive home support (Clarke et al., 2020). This was noted over a few years, providing evidence that these services need time to mature. But let us take this back to our person living with complex needs and examine the difference for Howard, whose time with the complex care team made a large difference to his life. When you consider integration of services that a complex care team allows, you can see that moves up from the person-focused care realm into functional integration, within normative integration and improving the ability of organisations to work together in a meaningful way for that person.

Chapter summary

In this chapter, we have explored how the context and interactions between different factors matters when it comes to those living with complex care needs. What this shows is that these laws, policies and procedures have an individual impact on every person who uses the health and social care system but particularly on those with complex needs. These factors may often be the cause of the issues the person is facing; secondary issues caused by medication make balancing their needs harder, and funding changes make the systems harder to navigate. The political matters on every level, and the cultural changes create tensions between groups. Prevention is made more difficult if you must choose between control of symptoms and the risk of diabetes or other conditions.

Socioeconomic status impacts the risk of multiple conditions. Complex needs do not exist in isolation, but in a network of related issues that either worsen the situation or ease it. If we as nurses are to strive towards supporting and advocating for our patients in the future, we must understand that.

Activities: brief outline answers

Activity 2.1 Critical thinking (page 23)

Consider Marmot's statistic around choice. What other determinants of health might prevent people from making choices?

If only one third of health is caused by traditional, biological risk factors, then two thirds are caused by the social and political determinants of health. You might have included poverty, social status, demographic, stress levels, life experiences, housing or disability.

Activity 2.2 Critical thinking (page 23)

The primary social determinants of health would include housing, disability and isolation.

Activity 2.3 Critical thinking (page 26)

You might have considered including inequalities, demographics, advocacy and economics. Within the adapted model, you could include the social determinants that impacted his life.

Activity 2.6 Team working (page 33)

- Howard's needs crossed several organisations and services, and his frequent admissions to hospital made it likely that he would be identified as complex. He was being contacted by housing, social services and healthcare services but was rejecting these.
- Howard was relocated to a new flat, which was on the ground floor, and linked into groups to give him social contact. His multiple healthcare needs and medications were reviewed, and

he was supported to take the medications he truly needed, with a number of them being stopped. He was supported and encouraged to accept help with cleaning and personal care.

- The social prescriber, the matron and the social worker were all involved. They worked with the healthcare team, housing and social services.
- They would need to share information with the GP, the county council, secondary care, housing and others.

Annotated further reading

lderwick, H., Dunn, P., McKenna, H., Walsh, N. and Ham, C. (2016) *Sustainability and Transformation Plans in the NHS*. London: King's Fund.

This document provides some background reading on the changes in the NHS, which will help you see the broader picture.

Cheng, C., Inder, K. and Chan, S.W.C. (2019) Patients' experiences of coping with multiple chronic conditions: a meta-ethnography of qualitative work. *International Journal of Mental Health Nursing*, 28(1), 54–70.

This article provides you a viewpoint from the patient's experiences. Understanding the lived experience of people in the situation allows you to better grasp their needs and your role in their lives.

Mullainathan, S. and Shafir, E. (2013) *Scarcity: Why Having Too Little Means So Much*. London: Times Books.

This book will give you some insights on the impact of poverty on the lives of people as well as the role 'busyness' has on our lives.

Useful websites

https://www.who.int/health-topics/social-determinants-of-health

This site provides background information on the social determinants of health, which play into every aspect of healthcare.

https://evidence.nihr.ac.uk/collection/making-sense-of-the-evidence-multiple-long-term-conditions-multimorbidity/

This collection of literature provides you with some help in exploring the issue of multi-morbidity.

Chapter 3 Socioeconomics in complex care

Chapter aims

After reading this chapter, you will be able to:

- understand the impact of the benefit system on claimants
- discuss the disability price tag
- understand the impact of socioeconomics on the lives of people with complex care needs.

Introduction

In the previous chapter, we looked at the broader context of living with complex care, including political and sociological determinants of health, policies and procedures. Let us now explore some of those in action and the impact that they can have. In this chapter, we will look at the benefit system in the UK and the impact that has on people with complex conditions. We will explore the disability price tag and the other socio-economic factors that impact on a person living with complexity.

We know that the higher the socioeconomic status a person holds, the lower the prevalence of health problems, illness, disease and death (Alvarez-Galvez, 2016). This relationship works both ways – the worse the health problems, the greater the impact on a person's socioeconomic status. Their findings made it clear that, in the UK, income is a major factor in determining health status. There are many ways to look at socioeconomics and complex needs; we could consider the cost-per-case to the NHS, the disability price tag, the cost burden to the country or many others. Let us start by putting a person at the heart of this discussion and explore the story that Bettie shared with us, before broadening our view.

Case study: Bettie

This is written from Bettie's point of view, in her own words.

When it became clear that I could no longer work in my career as a nurse, a profession that I had worked hard at for over 22 years, I was devastated. I was exhausted though, having suffered from a breakdown and ending up in a psychiatric hospital. Working as a practice sister at the same practice where I was a patient was not without problems and I was under pressure from my employers to return to work following my breakdown. When I saw my GP for appointments regarding my mental health, they were unable to see me as a patient with needs. Instead, they saw me as a member of their team that they could no longer be without. Something had to give and that was me, but without my income and with a family to support I was faced with having to see if I was eligible to claim a benefit. The form was several pages long and

(Continued)

(Continued)

required me to go into details about why I couldn't work, what symptoms I had and how they affected me. I felt on trial and it was like reliving all my painful, traumatic experiences again.

I knew I had done nothing wrong in the past to put me in this position, and I knew I was doing nothing wrong by seeking help from the system that I had been paying into for years yet I still felt guilty.

Luckily, I was successful in my claim for Employment and Support Allowance but after a year I was called into the Benefits Office for them to see me physically and assess my claim. I felt yet again that I was being judged and not believed.

Even now, every time the post drops through the letterbox I expect to see a letter informing me that my benefits have been stopped.

In this scenario, we can see how easily someone can go from a stable financial position, in work, to struggling financially. We can see the emotions entangled in the act of claiming the benefits people are entitled to and how complex the system itself is.

Activity 3.1   Critical thinking

Take a moment to reflect on the story Bettie shared with us. Consider the impact it might have to work in a job you love and experience what she did. Consider then the pressure of attempting to fill in the forms, to claim an income, while you are unwell.

As this activity is based on your own thoughts, no outline answer is given at the end of this chapter.

Day and Shaw (2020) found that there were themes of fear and trepidation for people living on benefits, and the impact of the media's narrative of 'scroungers' feeding into more stigma and people's own issues with identifying as disabled to claim benefits. Add to that the challenges of navigating a system that is complex and has a reputation for requiring people applying for PIP to go to appeal to be successful and you can see why it may be daunting.

The UK benefit system

We discussed this a little in Chapter 2, but here we will focus on PIP. It replaced the Disability Living Allowance (DLA) but was changed in 2017, amid great protest from patient groups such as the MS Society, Parkinson's UK and Mind. In Scotland, PIP was replaced by the Adult Disability Payment (ADP) in 2021, with fewer face-to-face assessments planned and with considerable consultation with people who have been through the PIP process as part of the design. PIP is meant to provide support with extra costs of living with a disability or long-term condition. Employment and Support Allowance (ESA) is to provide money for people who cannot work; this requires a work capability assessment (WCA).

The face-to-face assessments are seen as being too technical, with little humanity and claimants feeling disrespected and a lack of understanding; the narrative in the papers of 'scroungers' and the impact of this assessment dehumanised people (Day and Shaw, 2020). Statistics from the Tribunal Service show that 73 per cent of appeals for PIP and ESA overturn the original denial of benefits for the claimant and that claimants received a better award. The appeals process requires the person to have the knowledge and energy to do it; this is a complex system and the challenge of appealing may be difficult without support. The time permitted to return the form, four weeks, was too short; many found they could not get the evidence or that they needed help to complete the long, complex form (MS Society, 2019).

Box 3.1   Appeal success rates for individual benefits

- Employment and Support Allowance (ESA): 77 per cent
- Personal Independence Payment (PIP): 76 per cent
- Disability Living Allowance (DLA): 69 per cent
- Universal Credit (UC): 61 per cent

At the level of appeals there is an expectation that when you apply for a benefit you will have to either prepare in advance to defend it or find the energy and resources to do so. This might mean ordering notes and searching for evidence to provide or asking those providing your care for supporting letters. You may need to find the financial resources to survive until those benefits are granted.

One important fact to know is that these benefits are gateways to other financial supports, such as Carer's Allowance and the Motability scheme. In addition, there is the risk of sanctions (a fine or cancellation of benefits). Of those people who responded to Mind's survey, 10 per cent had been sanctioned; 89 per cent of those threatened with sanctions had worsened mental health (Mind, 2017).

Activity 3.2   Reflection

Pause here for a moment and reflect on your income, or that of your family. What would happen if you became too ill to work tomorrow? Go the benefit pages and work out which benefits you would claim, how and whether that would cover the costs of your living (including emergencies such as a car or washing machine break down).

As this activity is based on your own thoughts, no outline answer is given at the end of this chapter.

The Vimes 'boots' index

An author once had a character express frustration at economic imbalances:

> *The reason that the rich were so rich, Vimes reasoned, was because they managed to spend less money.*
>
> *Take boots, for example. He earned thirty-eight dollars a month plus allowances. A really good pair of leather boots cost fifty dollars. But an affordable pair of boots, which were sort of OK for a season or two and then leaked like hell when the cardboard gave out, cost about ten dollars. [...] But the thing was that good boots lasted for years and years. A man who could afford fifty dollars had a pair of boots that'd still be keeping his feet dry in ten years' time, while the poor man who could only afford cheap boots would have spent a hundred dollars on boots in the same time and would still have wet feet.*
>
> *This was the Captain Samuel Vimes 'Boots' theory of socioeconomic unfairness.*
>
> (Pratchett, 2013, p. 35)

Jack Monroe used this to illustrate her discussion on the consumer price index (which includes the price of champagne), highlighting the change in the poorest end of the market compared to the more expensive end. That is a poverty price tag, and when we bring it back to our people living with complex needs we investigate the disability price tag.

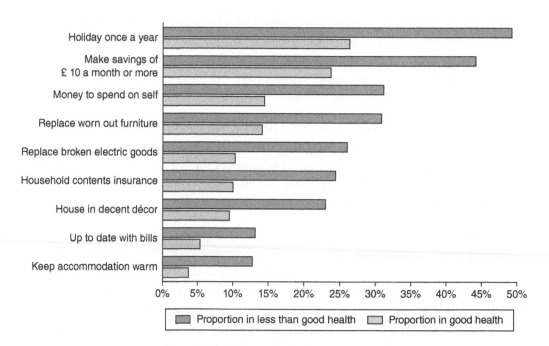

Figure 3.1   Material deprivation (The King's Fund, 2021)

The disability price tag

Living with disability costs more, increasing inequality; the disability price tag *is the additional monthly income a disabled person would need in order to enjoy the same standard of living as a non-disabled person* (Scope, 2019). This is around £583 a month, rising to more than £1000 for one in five. One in four families face that extra £1000 a month. If you look at Figure 3.1 you can see that the longer lines (those in less than good health) are less likely to be able to afford different items or services.

The term used by The King's Fund is 'material deprivation', which means when someone cannot afford necessities (The King's Fund, 2021). Look at the bottom of Figure 3.1; 13 per cent of people in the study were not able to afford to keep their home warm, three times higher than those in good health, before the cost-of-living crisis.

Activity 3.3 Reflection

The inability to pay for basic needs to be met, such as utility bills, is a massive barrier to health and well-being. A person living with a respiratory condition may risk worsening of their condition, leading to infection and admission, should their home be insufficiently heated. A person with poor mobility may fall and remain on the floor for a long period of time, risking pneumonia.

Building on Activity 3.2, reflect on the outcome of that if you were living with a complex need.

As this activity is based on your own thoughts, no outline answer is given at the end of this chapter.

In the most deprived of Scotland's population, life expectancies are thirteen years shorter for men and nine years for women compared to the most affluent areas. Other literature supports this finding that deprived people spend more time in poor health before death than the higher areas of affluence (Barnett et al., 2012; Scottish Government, 2020). Multi-morbidity is strongly linked to socioeconomic deprivation (Joseph Rowntree Foundation, 2015); the poorer you are, the more likely you are to be dealing with the issues we have discussed, struggling to pay bills and keep houses warm.

The impact this has on families who have children with complex needs is demonstrated well by Woodgate et al. (2015) (see Chapter 10). You can see that holidays, social life, work and couples time all become less likely. This study did not only include socioeconomic factors in the cause of these differences, but the link is two-way – it is more expensive to have complexity in your life and you are less likely to be able to work. This may mean that the parents need to consider the work they can do, such as Rosemary and her son Harry.

Activity 3.4   Critical thinking

Rosemary and Harry

You previously met Rosemary and Harry, a young boy with haemophilia. One of the primary risks for people with haemophilia is that of a bleed. This varies in significance – a bleed into a joint is exceptionally painful, whereas a bleed into the skull may be fatal. As a family, they decided that Harry would not be restricted in his activities by his condition, and he takes part in martial arts and other exercise activities.

If a bleed occurs, it is vital to take him to the specialist treatment centre an hour away as soon as possible; this may happen regularly. Rosemary and her husband must have a plan for one of them to leave and take him to the hospital at a moment's notice.

What impact might this have on Rosemary's employment? What contingency planning may they have to do for both parents to work?

A brief outline is provided at the end of the chapter.

Having an employer who is tolerant of their employees leaving their workplace abruptly like that on a regular basis is unlikely. Although the law says that employers should do all they can do to support someone to get back to work, it informs them that they can fire someone if they cannot do their job because there are no reasonable adjustments (UK Government, n.d.). Although Rosemary is lucky in that she is educated, in a profession that allows the flexibility and employed by an organisation that can adapt should she need to leave, many are not.

Impact

Now we know that people living in deprivation are more likely to have complexity, people with poor health are less likely to be able to cover essentials such as heating and bills and this extends to parenting a child with complex needs.

Broadening the view again, let's look at the impact of this in relation to things such as hospital admissions; people with lower incomes are more likely to be readmitted to hospital within the next year, and length of stay and chances of dying are higher than those with better incomes (Schjødt et al., 2019). This was in a similar system to the UK (the person getting the prescription must pay a fee); people with lower incomes were less likely to get their prescriptions filled.

Although this information relates to all long-term conditions, it impacts those living with complex conditions; the mismatch between the way our society operates and their needs becomes set in stark relief here, where basic needs such as food, housing, etc. are not available without great stress. We are frequently told that long-term conditions are a 'tsunami', worsened by the impact of the pandemic, structural racism and determinants of health (Califf, 2021). The upstream decisions made by those in the room when policies are formed impact every aspect of life.

Cost to the NHS or social care of an individual with multi-morbidity, which many people living with complexity experience, is no different to having two people, with one condition. In fact, Adomako-Mensah et al. (2020) found that there is a reduction in cost. They suggest that this may be because the person can be seen in a single appointment, reducing costs compared to two people having two appointments. Another possibility is that care is overlapping or inadequate; the lack of joined up care between mental and physical health is a major issue for people living with complexity – they often experience both, with the likelihood of mental health problems rising the more physical health issues a person has (Barnett et al., 2012), and we think this is likely to be true for the reverse, since mental health is often linked with a reduction in physical health. This is more likely in deprived areas than in more affluent areas.

Cost-effective systems

So let us look a little into what cost-effective systems mean.

There are different measures: cost analysis, cost utility analysis, cost–benefit analysis and cost-effectiveness analysis. Each compares the benefits of an intervention with the costs, but with different measurements of the outcomes of that. Cost analysis measures costs in money. Cost utility analysis uses health state preference scores such as healthy years or quality-adjusted life years. Cost–benefit analysis uses money vs outcomes. Cost-effectiveness analysis looks at one consequence, and how effective the activity is compared to the alternatives – it may measure years of life gained, quality-adjusted life years, diagnosis made, blood pressure reduction, cholesterol change and so on (Drummond et al., 2015). This can be found in much of the medical literature – that is, randomised controlled trials.

NICE definition of quality-adjusted life year

A measure of the state of health of a person or group in which the benefits, in terms of length of life, are adjusted to reflect the quality of life. One quality-adjusted life year (QALY) is equal to one year of life in perfect health, calculated by estimating the years of life remaining for a patient following a particular treatment or intervention and weighting each year with a quality-of-life score (on a 0 to 1 scale). It is often measured in terms of the person's ability to carry out the activities of daily life, and freedom from pain and mental disturbance (National Institute for Health and Care Excellence, n.d.)

This measure of cost-effectiveness can either be used to inform coverage decisions or ration care (deciding what care is provided or not) but it always is used to influence the choice of activities that make good use of resources. This might be preventative medicine (cervical smears, vaccination programmes or testing); it is commonly used by

NICE, and they have a clear aim to maximise health gain with limited resources (Cylus et al., 2016).

It is common to use bed-days saved within the NHS: how many of these units can be saved by prevention of an admission by a team. It is vital to remember that the outcome we measure becomes the target those within the service will aim for. You can take the four-hour rule from emergency care as an example of this; a more nuanced rule that meets the needs for more urgent conditions such as sepsis may be a more useful active measurement and driver (Campbell et al., 2017).

In comparing healthcare systems, you often see the comparison of how much of the gross domestic product was spent on health compared to how much death rates decreased. Studies have shown that the NHS is a system that has good cost-effectiveness compared to others, such as the US (Pritchard and Wallace, 2011).

Complex care teams and services

Relating that back to our people living with complexity, you can see the drivers for the creation of teams working to support them within the community and preventing unnecessary admissions. The need to access certain skills and for professionals to work through the barriers to integration of health and social care is vital.

Case study: Bettie

The complex care team received a referral for Bettie. She had multiple health conditions including diabetes, cataracts, leg ulcers, thrush and obesity. Bettie was struggling to manage her activities of daily living (ADLs) and was regularly missing medical appointments. Bettie struggled to clean her home, which was becoming very untidy, dirty and had cat faeces and urine on the floor. She spent most of the time in bed in her lounge.

Activity 3.5   Critical thinking

Consider which skills and professionals might be useful to Bettie's case?

A brief outline is provided at the end of the chapter.

Nursing and cost-effectiveness

The NMC has argued that investment in nursing is a path to more cost-effectiveness in our healthcare system (Crisp et al., 2018). Certainly, in preventative medicine with screening and health promotion nursing holds a central role. Crisp and colleagues speak about universal healthcare and the fact that is vital in helping people to live healthy lives and experience well-being, alongside the benefits to global health security and epidemic preparedness, something we have experienced in the pandemic.

Money is not the sole driver in care, but it can cause considerable harm to both individuals and communities of patients. You can explore many well-known scandals but the Contaminated Blood Scandal or Death by Indifference are good places to start since they demonstrate the role healthcare professionals can play in this harm, for good or bad (Haemophilia Society, n.d.; UK Government, 2013; Mencap, 2012).

Case study: Michael

Michael is twenty years old. He has a diagnosis of severe learning disabilities, autism and epilepsy and has two to three tonic-clonic seizures per week. Michael lives in a residential care home with five other people with learning disabilities in a modern housing estate. He attends a day centre in his local area and travels there in a minibus with eleven other 'clients'. He is in a class with ten other pupils with varying levels of learning and physical disability, all of whom use verbal language and communication. One student in the class has short but noisy outbursts at least once a day, occasionally with physical violence directed at other students and staff (staff have relevant training to support with this).

Michael speaks in short sentences, mainly in response to a request or command, and occasionally when he asks for someone or something. He can read and write a few simple words, count to twenty and has some numeracy skills. He recognises money and knows that notes (£5, £10, etc.) are 'bigger' than coins, but struggles with recognising correct change. Michael chooses his own clothes, but they are often considered 'too old' and formal for him. He buys them with the support of his key worker, Freda, who is 58 years old and has known him since he was a baby.

Michael speaks very loudly, appearing to derive pleasure from the sensation. Michael will jump and spin around, and flaps his hands, sometimes letting out a high-pitched cry, which he seems to enjoy the sensation of. Michael likes to sit on swings in a playground, appearing to enjoy the sensory experience. Occasionally, Michael's behaviour can escalate into an outburst including screaming and breaking things, but he has never been violent towards others. Staff have training to support him at these times.

Michael's behaviours are more likely to escalate if he is tired (sometimes he does not sleep at night), and either just before or after an epileptic seizure (unless he sleeps after it). Michael likes to spend time on his own and can withdraw from group activities in the day centre. He likes to keep things organised and tidy, and his clothes and possessions are neatly categorised and kept in their place.

(Continued)

(Continued)

Michael takes time to get used to new, busy, bustling and noisy environments, or other people who are noisy and rushing around, but can do so with support and time. Michael does not like to be touched very much, although he will accept a firm hand on his arm or elbow to guide him somewhere if he knows and trusts the person. Michael likes Kylie Minogue videos and music, and he loves Harry Potter, including looking at books and magazines, and on film. Michael responds well to routine and structure, liking familiar activities and people.

Michael has limited contact with his family (occasional visits from a brother), but he does have some people who are important in his life and that he responds to positively:

- Freda, his key worker;
- Kevin, a community Learning Disabilities Nurse, who has known him for a long time and sees Michael three or four times a year for updates, reviews and general contact;
- Bob, who was a key worker for Michael when he was young and first came into services in short-term (respite) care and as a young man in residential services. Bob has stayed in contact with Michael over the years and visits to take him out about once a month. He attends review meetings and acts as an official advocate for Michael in meetings. Michael loves Bob and is at his most relaxed, friendly and communicative when he is with Bob.

Activity 3.6   Decision-making

Working with people with complex needs means that we should make reasonable adjustments to adapt our methods of delivering healthcare to their individual requirements. Consider Michael's case study, and reflect on the adjustments you might have to make in your treatment with them? How would you know they needed them?

A brief outline answer is given at the end of the chapter.

Countering health disparities

Within our healthcare system, despite it being universal healthcare, free at the point of contact, there remain inequalities and disparities. We can see this in problems that are not addressed in national policie; Salway et al. (2020) highlight the risk of hepatitis B in people who migrated from East Asia, or safeguarding legislation in female genital mutilation, which has increased negative stereotyping of the Somali community in some regions of the UK. Even basics such as oral health can be an area where health disparities can be found; people with learning disabilities have a higher prevalence of oral health issues (Wilson et al., 2019). Throughout the healthcare system, examples of inequalities can be found. Remember the inequalities and disability price tag for people who live with complexity and that they are more likely to experience deprivation already.

As nurses, we need to be aware of the impact of this on our patients; in complexity, people are more likely to be affected by these issues. McFarland and MacDonald (2019) put this firmly in the realm of nursing responsibilities – providing health education, promoting health and recovery, and supporting health protection. We work on the front line in every aspect of healthcare, providing holistic care in almost every circumstance a human may find themselves in, from before birth to death. Working in this role with people living with complexity in their lives requires us to work as part of a team to tackle that disparity and inequality on an individual and population level. Being aware of the resources available to our patients and advocating for further support for them are key aspects for us as nurses. We must balance this advocacy for our patients in our area with an awareness of the impact of unequal and inaccessible services when compared across the UK. We can advocate for policy change, taking leadership roles from politics to roles within organisations such as NHS England, Public Health England and the World Health Organization.

Chapter summary

Let us think back to Bettie and Rosemary; consider how socioeconomics impact their lives. Bettie's fight with the benefit system was a challenge she chose to share with us all. Rosemary, whose son accesses a specialist unit, is lucky enough to have a job that can be flexible for when she must take him there for his routine emergency care.

On every level in the lives of people with complexity, socioeconomics plays a part, one that cannot be overlooked and should be addressed by nurses who care for them.

Activities: brief outline answers

Activity 3.4 Critical thinking (page 42)

Rosemary and Harry

Rosemary was lucky that she had an employer who could, most of the time, manage her need to leave abruptly. In certain professions this is possible but in many it is not. In shift work, for example, leaving frequently without warning may have a catastrophic impact on employment.

Her husband adapted his working hours, so he was able to do the same on certain days of the week. She enrolled her family in the plan, arranging for car seats to be in three family member's cars so that any one of them was prepared to take him to the specialist centre. This did happen several times.

Because Harry is not an only child, this departure for the specialist centre required someone to be available to care for his sibling, who may need picking up from school.

Activity 3.5 Critical thinking (page 44)

The ability of the full extended MDT team to make the connection and support her in making choices around her needs and engagement with the team is vital. They would be able to assess all health and social needs, and act as a multidisciplinary team. By design, they work across organisational boundaries. With the issues she has, she could have ended up being admitted to a hospital or to a care home. Bettie herself was clear that she wished to remain in her home, and several actions were taken to ensure that was the case.

Adaptions within her house allowed her to manage with a small care package that the team arranged. In addition, the team prioritised her wish to communicate with her family more easily, obtaining a laptop through a grant and arranging lessons for her to learn how to use it.

Activity 3.6 Decision-making (page 46)

Potential adjustments for Michael in healthcare interactions:

- extra time for appointments;
- appointments at quiet times;
- pre-appointment visits to services to get used to the environment and people;
- consistent/repeated staff;
- appointments at home if possible;
- visual aids, such as 'objects of reference', pictures, 'social stories' (see Chapter 9);
- include a sensory experience that calms Michael and may help him engage in a consultation or conversation such as swinging, or accepting that he may make high-pitched sounds to calm himself;
- include a consistent, familiar member of Michael's support team in appointment to help him manage it;
- awareness training for your staff about autism, complex and challenging behaviours and learning disabilities.

How do you know you need to make these adjustments?

We suggest:

- thorough and individualised assessment processes to understand and meet Michael's needs;
- multidisciplinary team working to obtain full information from a range of professionals who know Michael well;
- involving Michael's family and other carers in discussions and care planning to ensure a fully rounded picture of him;
- developing a strong, positive values base towards people with learning disabilities and autism, and promoting inclusion and individualised care will ensure this becomes embedded in your care practice.

Annotated further reading

Day, W. and Shaw, R. (2020) When benefit eligibility and patient-led care intersect. Living in the UK with chronic illness: experiences of the work capability assessment. *Journal of Health Psychology*, 135910532095347.

This study demonstrated that capturing the experience of people in situations like this is vital to understanding what is happening.

Crisp, N., Brownie, S. and Refsum, C. (2018) Nursing and midwifery: the key to the rapid and cost-effective expansion of high quality universal healthcare. *Doha, Qatar, World Innovation Summit for Health,* 1–39.

This report gives a thoughtful view from nursing and is worth a full read.

Useful websites

https://www.kingsfund.org.uk/publications/what-are-health-inequalities

This site provides a thoughtful view on health inequalities, among other issues. They tend to be evidence-based and balanced in their approach.

https://www.countyhealthrankings.org/explore-health-rankings/measures-data-sources/county-health-rankings-model/health-factors/social-and-economic-factors

This page allows you to explore the issues in more depth, providing information from the world.

Chapter 4 Strategies in complex care

NMC Future Nurse: Standards of Proficiency for Registered Nurses

This chapter will address the following platforms and proficiencies:

Platform 1: Being an accountable professional

1.3   understand and apply the principles of courage, transparency and the professional duty of candour, recognising and reporting any situations, behaviours or errors that could result in poor care outcomes

1.5   understand the demands of professional practice and demonstrate how to recognise signs of vulnerability in themselves or their colleagues and the action required to minimise risks to health

1.8   demonstrate the knowledge, skills and ability to think critically when applying evidence and drawing on experience to make evidence informed decisions in all situations

1.9   understand the need to base all decisions regarding care and interventions on people's needs and preferences, recognising and addressing any personal and external factors that may unduly influence their decisions

1.10 demonstrate resilience and emotional intelligence and be capable of explaining the rationale that influences their judgements and decisions in routine, complex and challenging situations

1.11 communicate effectively using a range of skills and strategies with colleagues and people at all stages of life and with a range of mental, physical, cognitive and behavioural health challenges

1.12 demonstrate the skills and abilities required to support people at all stages of life who are emotionally or physically vulnerable

1.13 demonstrate the skills and abilities required to develop, manage and maintain appropriate relationships with people, their families, carers and colleagues

1.14 provide and promote non-discriminatory, person-centred and sensitive care at all times, reflecting on people's values and beliefs, diverse backgrounds, cultural characteristics, language requirements, needs and preferences, taking account of any need for adjustments

1.17 take responsibility for continuous self-reflection, seeking and responding to support and feedback to develop their professional knowledge and skills

Platform 2: Promoting health and preventing ill health

2.1 understand and apply the aims and principles of health promotion, protection and improvement and the prevention of ill health when engaging with people

Platform 3: Assessing needs and planning care

3.1 demonstrate and apply knowledge of human development from conception to death when undertaking full and accurate person-centred nursing assessments and developing appropriate care plans

3.2 demonstrate and apply knowledge of body systems and homeostasis, human anatomy and physiology, biology, genomics, pharmacology and social and behavioural sciences when undertaking full and accurate person-centred nursing assessments and developing appropriate care plans

Platform 6: Improving safety and quality of care

6.11 acknowledge the need to accept and manage uncertainty, and demonstrate an understanding of strategies that develop resilience in self and others

Chapter aims

After reading this chapter, you will be able to:

- understand the principles of the nursing process as it relates to the care of people with complex needs
- demonstrate an understanding of the use of self as a therapeutic tool and how to care for yourself to do this safely
- understand the principles and processes in planning care with people with complex needs.

Introduction

As nurses, we are often in the home of a person living with complexity, and often involved in their care. In this chapter, we will explore the issues within complex care around goal setting, applying the nursing process and collaborative care. We consider the issues with measurement of outcomes and benchmarking when the objectives and options are unknown or uncertain. We will discuss the nurse as a therapeutic tool in practice.

The nursing process

The nursing process originated from the US, moving to the UK in the 1980s (Peate, 2019). It is designed to establish a systemic process to provide nursing care, moving through a cycle of assessment, nursing diagnosis, planning and delivering care, and reviewing the outcomes. Simply put, the nursing process is a way of organising work-load and the tasks within that workload to ensure that all the patient's needs are met. It should be a systemic review of the situation, forming a plan and then reviewing the plan – in a very similar way to the scientific method used in research – completed alongside the patient and the rest of the team.

One model that is related to the nursing process is the Roper–Logan–Tierney model of nursing (Figure 4.1); this produced a list of twelve activities of daily living (ADLs) which nurses can use to help guide their assessments and care plans (Williams, 2017). These activities are part of being human, from birth to the grave, and complex care needs impact on people's ability to perform them independently. You can see how that may interact with the nursing process; using those ADLs to view the whole of a person's life is useful if it does not become a 'tick box' process.

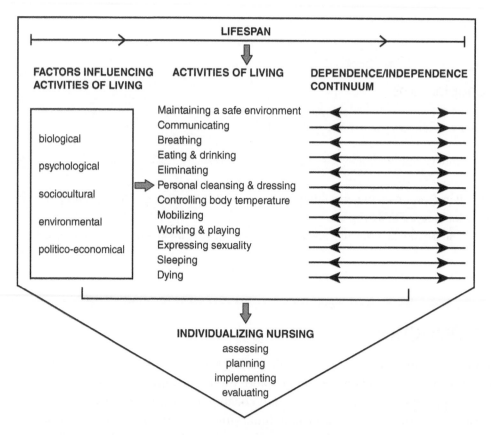

Figure 4.1 Roper–Logan–Tierney model of nursing (Roper, 1996)

There are a few barriers to implementing this approach – not least that our health service is built around acute episodes of care, even with general practice, where you have incidental interactions when required. Zheng et al. (2019) identified several barriers in their study, which ranged from organisational ability to change to the economic status of the patient, early discharges, lack of cooperation and the level of knowledge within the staff. They found that the more stressful the location, the less likely it was that the nursing process would be used; the more knowledgeable the nurse, the more likely they would use it; and the economic status of the patient correlated clearly – the poorer the patient, the less likely they were to have the nursing process involved in their care. This study was undertaken in the US, where a large part of their healthcare requires funding; despite this, you can see echoes of it within the UK's need to pay for prescriptions or home care. These barriers are found in a study by Zamanzadeh et al. (2015) in Iran; they found that, alongside those barriers, the lack of understanding of the nursing process featured heavily in the barriers. They suggest that increasing knowledge and awareness are vital to improving this.

Case study: Isabella

Isabella is a 58-year-old lady with an unidentified neurodegenerative disorder (sometimes neurological conditions don't always fit a diagnosis we recognise). She lives at home with her wife and is supported there by a 24-hour care package. Due to her condition, she does not have capacity to make decisions related to her care, and the team rely on her advance care plans and her advocate in the form of her wife.

Her care team include a specialist neurological team, her GP, the community nurses, the nurses and carers from the care package provider, her pharmacist, speech and language therapist, physiotherapist and occupational therapist.

Assessments are a vital part of this process, the bedrock upon which the whole process is built. Gathering that information involves not only documentation and the healthcare team but also must include the person living with complexity. Critical thinking is vital as part of this process, and your assessment should include all aspects of someone's life – physical, emotional, spiritual, sexual, financial, cultural and cognitive – as it pertains to the role you are undertaking. People living with complex needs may already have experienced multiple assessments by many different professionals and teams, and their experiences will impact your interactions. This means that your care of them must differ from when you work with someone whose needs are relatively comparatively straightforward. Their experiences and knowledge should weigh more heavily in your thinking, and the interaction you have must consider the potential traumatic experiences they may have been through.

Activity 4.1   Reflection

Considering Isabella's situation, what experiences would you wish to have considered when you think about your own needs, if you were faced with needing this type of care? How many assessments would you be willing to repeat the same information for?

As this is based on your own reflection, no outline answer is provided at the end of this chapter.

Trauma-informed care

Thompson-Lastad et al. (2017) cited a presenter at a complex care management conference as saying, *What if we approached all care assuming that everyone has been exposed to trauma?* and that is the approach we will take in this book – that all of those living with complex needs have had that potential trauma in their lives. We know that chronic stress and trauma are linked with changes in health, and we have discussed the issues around that in Chapters 2 and 3. Thompson-Lastad et al. (2017) note the broad range of literature that supports the higher-than-average levels of trauma in people with complex care needs. Trauma-informed care has four attributes; recognition, knowledge, concern and respect (Guest, 2021) (see Figure 4.2).

Case study: Bettie

Commentary in her own words.

I have yet to encounter any professional, let alone a nurse who has appeared to take into account my previous traumatic experiences. I particularly remember one nurse who dismissed my trauma, dismissed my distress and dismissed my fears. Her treatment of me bordered on cruelty and I will forever remember her name. In my experience areas from this model particularly lacking have been shared decision-making, honesty and promoting and safeguarding the trust of those affected by trauma.

In the study by Thompson-Lastad et al. (2017), they spoke with two complex care management (CCM) teams in the US and explored the way the staff discuss the trauma their patients experience, and how that allows them to understand the context of the patients' lives. It explored the disconnect from CCM programmes and the needs of the people living with complex needs. From this study, the frequently short interventions of CCM programmes (discussed more in Chapter 5) are often worked around by staff members who use the flexibility of the programmes to work more broadly on the systemic issues the patient is facing; they can spend more time with patients and be more flexible around the appointments themselves. They used a slower approach to build relationships with the person, despite the pressure of the CCM programme design which is built around reducing hospitalisation for this group of patients.

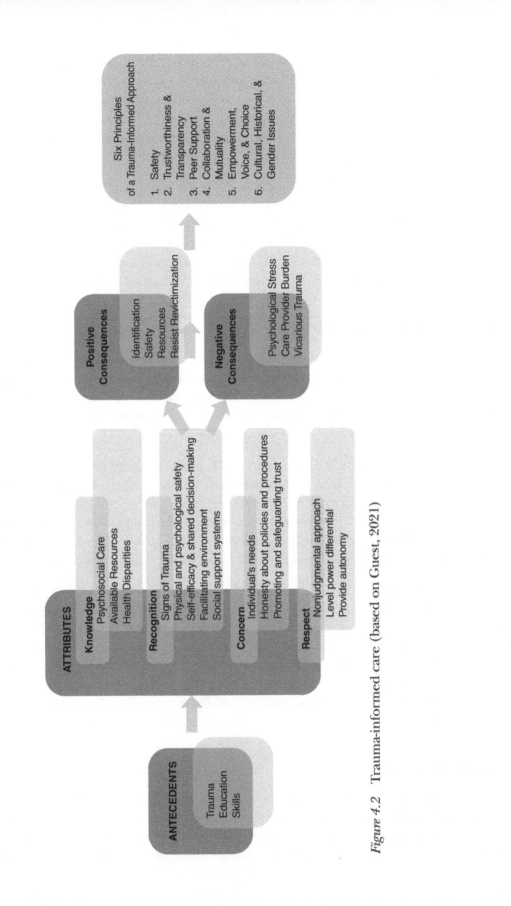

Figure 4.2 Trauma-informed care (based on Guest, 2021)

One key finding from the Thompson-Lastad et al. study (2017) was that naming trauma allows us to name the structural issues that cause the trauma in a way that makes it clear to the patient and those around us that one of the true needs is to combat the existing inequity. This is echoed in the work by Guest (2021), who identified that trauma-informed care results in the ability to identify the people with trauma, safety for those around them, increased access of resources and avoiding repeating the harm.

This approach has been more common within mental health and Learning Disability Nursing, and Isobel and Edwards (2017) describe the processes and effects of implementing this trauma-informed care (TIC) model of care on an acute ward in Sydney, in a health system like the UK. The definition of TIC they used considered the need for emotional and psychological safety, alongside awareness of the impact of the trauma and the person's experiences of care (more on this in Chapters 8, 9 and 10).

Impact on the clinician

Managing your own behaviours and needs is a vital part of trauma-informed care. Guest (2021) found that staff experienced vicarious trauma after hearing the experiences of their patients. We know that we use our therapeutic relationships to help our patients, and in that we use ourselves as a therapeutic tool by the conscious use of our personality, judgements and perceptions to help them (Yazdani et al., 2021).

Kwaitek et al. (2005) spoke about the impact our own attribution (meanings we give to something that happens) have on our behaviour and practice. In Learning Disability Nursing and mental health particularly, behaviours that challenge us can find us attributing intent or purpose that may not exist. Therefore, reflective practice is vital – pausing to consider the biases and beliefs that are acting on the interaction provides opportunities to explore their experience in that moment in a more helpful, considered way.

Your own experiences bring bias and beliefs to the interaction; in nursing, some may use self-disclosure of their own experiences to help the relationship building (Steuber and Pollard, 2018). This can be a challenging thing to balance, without removing the focus from the patient and making the moment about you and your needs instead. The benefits may outweigh those risks if you have the skills to manage it; it may help humanising the relationship, reducing the power imbalance and placing you on the side of your patient during this journey. Steuber and Pollard (2018) identified the need for debriefing to support nurses with this practice and help us to manage our own emotions.

Managing self

Therapeutic use of self is a common and vital concept within all nursing roles; Koloroutis (2014) explored the capabilities that we need to manage that and allow ourselves to be part of the therapeutic process for our patients. She identified three: self-attunement, self-clarity and self-compassion. These practices are part of a mindful practice, which helps us to balance the needs of our patients, the use of our own selves as therapeutic tools and our own well-being. It gives us permission to show compassion to both our patients and ourselves; she gives examples of speaking kindly to yourself as you do this work, and reflectively considering your own beliefs.

Activity 4.2   Reflection

Consider the following reflections and write out your thoughts in your reflection journal.

- Who are the practitioners that I respect? What is it in their practices that make me feel like that?
- What information and knowledge do I need and how can I access that?
- Which patients do I find challenging, and how do I react?
- Which patients do I like, and what is it that makes their care enjoyable for me?
- What have my patients taught me?
- What is my nursing philosophy (i.e., what beliefs do you have that you hold in practice)?

As this activity is based on your own reflection, no outline answer is given at the end of this chapter.

You can see that our skills interact with our patients, the situations they are in and the constraints and benefits of our occupation. The latter relates to the scope of practice that is vital to our work. But it is important to remember that we are not working alone – we work collaboratively, with our patient and our colleagues. We may be working with people outside the health system, such as the work Harry's specialist nurse did with the school – the MDT, both in health and in other organisations, is vital. We are very rarely the only person involved (see Chapter 5).

Case study: Harry

Harry, our haemophiliac child, was about to start school. One issue that Rosemary faced was the knowledge that she or her husband would need to leave work abruptly whenever he sustained an injury, to take him to the specialist centre. Without the school having the expert knowledge they had built up around whether a bleed was urgent or not, they would be called to make that decision in the middle of their workday on the telephone.

Harry's specialist nurse reached out to the school with Rosemary's support and did an education session, working as a group to create a plan and guidelines so that there was a level of knowledge to support him there. That collaborative care, reaching outside the NHS to provide family-centred care, helped Harry and his family make the transition.

Activity 4.3   Critical thinking

Considering the scenario above, can you think about the broader implications of a child with complex needs attending school? Harry has a sibling, Hermione, who had not yet started school at that point, but you should include her in your thinking.

A brief outline answer is provided at the end of this chapter.

Collaborative care

There is a large amount of evidence supporting collaborative care in all fields of nursing (Bekelman et al., 2018; Camacho et al., 2018; Gilbody, 2006; Katon et al., 2010; Pfaff and Markaki, 2017; Talbott et al., 2021). In physical health conditions, such as heart failure, collaborative care around symptoms and psychosocial issues reduced the negative impacts, improving depression and fatigue in the patients (Bekelman et al., 2018). In mental health nursing, collaborative care reduced depression (see Chapter 7) (Camacho et al., 2018; Gilbody, 2006). People living with complexity often experience depression and chronic illness; Katon et al. (2010) found that collaborative care reduced cholesterol levels, blood pressure and depression scores. It improved quality of life and satisfaction with care. This is shown in young people with attention-deficit hyperactivity disorder, where collaboration between teams removed existing barriers between schools and healthcare, improving the support for the children and their families (Talbott et al., 2021).

Therefore, with this evidence in every field, it does seem logical that we should see collaborative care throughout the healthcare field. But is that the case?

Activity 4.4   Reflection

Think back to your last practice placement: what examples of collaborative care did you see there? Where did you see lost opportunities to restructure the healthcare your team was providing to make it more collaborative?

As this activity is based on your own reflection, no outline answer is given at the end of this chapter.

Within this book, we have spoken about the complex care team; their model of care is collaborative. This type of care service works across boundaries from health and social care, identifying barriers to the patient's needs and working around them. It is vital that, as we collaborate, the patient is part of that team. The work should not focus on the needs of the healthcare team or the system but the needs of the person at the heart of the process. One key factor in this is the setting of goals; when these are set, it is vital that we follow through on our promises and act.

Implementation

This stage involves putting the plan into action; this might be a nursing intervention in most literature (i.e., ECGs, oxygen, etc.), but in the context of complex care, it may be arrangements for care, financial support, equipment, access to services or housing adjustments (Toney-Butler and Thayer, 2020). Referrals to other services and collaboration within the multidisciplinary team are key to this stage.

Evaluation

This is vital, allowing the participants to reflect on the impact of the process; has it worked? Do we need to revisit and form a secondary plan? Since the lives of those living with complex needs are rarely straightforward and their needs evolve over time, it is unlikely a single cycle through the process would be sufficient.

Outcome measures can vary widely but using patient-reported outcome measures (PROMs) and patient-reported experience measures (PREMs) can be a way to continue the conversations that should have occurred throughout the nursing process. These are often questionnaires that measure the person's view of their health status or ones that measure their perceptions of their experience while receiving care (Kingsley and Patel, 2017).

PROMs should be standardised, validated tools that the person completes; it assesses their view of their health, impact on ADLs and quality of life and may be disease-specific or generic (Kingsley and Patel, 2017). PREMs gather information on the person's experience and are often questionnaires that explore communication or whether the care was timely. Not only are these useful for helping us have conversations and measure impact of our care but they can be used in research. It is vital that the right choice of tool is made to measure the outcome; using a tool that is not validated means it is not tested to measure the thing you want it to measure. You can see examples of this in Table 4.1. Kingsley and Patel (2017) note that there is a link between the experience and the outcomes.

PROMs	PREMs
Measuring service level quality of care (benchmarking)	Collecting feedback for healthcare staff on quality of care
Measuring efficacy of clinical interventions (randomised clinical trials)	Measuring effectiveness of the processes
Measuring cost-effectiveness (see NICE guidelines)	Gaining insight into the patient experience of your service
Clinical audit	Quality improvement of patient-centred care

Table 4.1 Uses for PROMs and PREMs

Activity 4.5   Reflection

Think back to your last practice placement: what tools did you see being used to assess clinical outcomes and patient experiences there? This might be something like NEWS2, Waterlow, or friends and family reporting.

As this activity is based on your own reflection, no outline answer is given at the end of this chapter.

PROMs should include the context of the situation, and decisions based on these should be made openly (Sawatzky et al., 2021). These PROMs can provide discussions around treatment options, new goals and continuation or addition of more services or support. The Working Group on Health Outcomes for Older Persons with Multiple Chronic Conditions (2012) produced some outcome measurement tools designed for use in older people with multiple chronic conditions; the things they measure would be beneficial to use in complex care. Measuring each of these areas may be completed with the appropriate validated tools.

Item	Purpose
General health	The self-perceived state of someone's health also should consider their knowledge and perceptions of their health. Their perception of their health might be wholly different to their healthcare team's perception
Symptom burden	Sometimes it is difficult to link a symptom with a particular condition, especially when you take a holistic view of health. However, you could then focus more on the symptoms that the person feels are the biggest problem for them and examine those in greater depth
Physical function and mobility	In complex care, this may be focused on ADLs, rather than the more specific gait speed-style questions
Mental health outcomes: mood and affect	Anxiety and depression are common in people living with complex care needs; from the conditions themselves and the situation they are in
Cognitive function	Memory, thought, perception, reasoning, orientation and behaviour changes over time. Dementia and delirium can be issues for people with complex needs and may be secondary to acute issues
Social health	Social support is a key issue for people with complex needs; factors that affect this are important in this area
Patient preferences and outcomes	Although the original working group identified this as a gap in their design, it is a vital part of complex care. The aims of the person with complex needs are key outcome measurements

Table 4.2   Measurements in complex care

Considerations for particular groups

When using PROMs and PREMs with groups, you must consider the accessibility needs of that group. This may look like providing privacy where the questions may cause distress, support to complete them, larger font sizes or more white space on the form (Jahagirdar et al., 2012). Being mindful of the emotional state and literacy levels of your patient is important since these assessments should avoid causing further distress and trauma whenever possible.

Limitations

Many of these tools are validated for research, not clinical practice, and therefore may not measure what we hope they might. They are language- and culture-specific, and validation needs to occur for each change of either of these (Kingsley and Patel, 2017).

Sawatzky et al. (2021) noted that, when using PROMs, you should be mindful of response shifts; this is when something has happened between our assessments that has changed the context of the conversation. This might be an acute episode for someone with chronic conditions or an intervention such as cognitive behavioural therapy changing the way the person thinks about their situation, for example. This can be used on a broader level, when considering service level agreements; for example, a response shift from a less inclusive and holistic concept of health such as a purely biological one to one that includes social well-being.

Chapter summary

The nursing process can give structure to the work you do with people with complex needs; it provides method in an area of practice in which the urgency of need can sometimes drive the situation. Ensuring that both your patient and you are safe when using your knowledge, experiences and personality as a therapeutic tool is a key aspect of care in this field. It is vital to keep the focus on the person throughout, centring both their needs and their experience of the care they receive.

In the next chapter, we will explore the way teams work within this field.

Activities: brief outline answers

Activity 4.3 Critical thinking (page 58)

The school would need to understand the risks and actions to take for a child who may experience consequences for falls. If an incident happens, there would need to be a clear plan for his journey to the specialist centre and for Hermione's collection from school. The school would need to know what is and is not an emergency, and have a clear plan around things like head injuries – they can hold medication and equipment to go in the ambulance with him, since local hospitals would not have his medication and equipment, reducing the risk of inhibitors. This would require equipment such as child seats; three members of their extended family kept child seats in their cars just in case this happened.

On days where he had routine treatments, he would miss school, so plans needed to be in place for him to catch up on his learning. Equally, since such occasions were framed as something fun with treats to reduce fear of the hospital, there would be a need to balance this for Hermione, so that she does not feel left out.

When considering holidays (if they can afford them), they need to consider where the closest specialist centre is. They cannot just leave him at a play place, and are only just letting him go on playdates without supervision. This could cause over-protective parenting for both children, since the rules must apply equally. He may find himself being treated differently by other children; this can raise issues of confidentiality. Access to school activities such as away days and camps can be problematic.

They should understand the parenting choices that Rosemary and Eddie have made so that the focus is family-centred care. It is vital that Hermione's needs are not subsumed in conversations with the family, since she deserves the same attention any other child would receive. Planning with the parents' workplaces is key, with some flexibility available for Rosemary to take Harry to planned and emergency appointments. Other family members have made space to do so, if necessary.

Annotated further reading

Toney-Butler, T. J. and Thayer, J. M. (2020) *Nursing Process.* San Francisco: StatPearls [Internet].

This article provides a basic description of the nursing process and we recommend it as a starting point.

Ead, H. (2019) Application of the nursing process in a complex health care environment. *Canadian Nurse.* https://www.canadian-nurse.com/blogs/cn-content/2019/09/16/application-of-the-nursing-process-in-a-complex-he

This article provides an illustration of the nursing process in action.

Moule, P., Armoogum, J., Douglass, E. and Taylor, J. (2017) Evaluation and its importance for nursing practice. *Nursing Standard,* 31(35), 55–63.

This article provides a thoughtful view on the importance of evaluation.

Useful websites

https://www.kingsfund.org.uk/publications/communities-and-health

The King's Fund provides a viewpoint of the importance of communities in health. In your assessment of your patient, you should consider the support they have around them.

http://careinfoscotland.scot/topics/how-to-get-care-services/hospital-based-complex-clinical-care/

This page demonstrates how people can access care services.

Chapter 5 — Multidisciplinary management

Chapter aims

After reading this chapter, you will be able to:

- understand the evidence behind multidisciplinary working
- be able to identify and discuss various models of care
- identify benefits and barriers to care coordination
- understand commissioning and integrated care systems.

Introduction

In the previous chapter, we focused on the strategies we can use and the impact of those (or the lack of them) on the people living with complex needs. In this chapter, we will explore the commissioning of services relevant to complex care, the models themselves and the issues in transitioning from one care system to another (i.e., from child to adult services).

The multidisciplinary team

To frame 'new' models of patient management, we should first be aware of the multidisciplinary team (MDT) and briefly look back at the issues that highlighted it as one of the solutions to problems in complex care management. You are likely aware that it generally consists of doctors, nurses, occupational therapists, physiotherapists, speech and language therapists, social workers and so on.

One way of exploring why MDTs became seen as a solution can be to look at where quality improvement methods have used data to highlight hotspots of problems for people with complex or long-term conditions. Gillespie and Reader (2018) spoke of patient-centred insights where complaints highlighted issues. These issues were primarily related to entering or exiting the healthcare system, whether that be a low-level problem or an omission. Clinical, relationship and management issues received a third of complaints each and a quarter had involved major harm. In this way, it is easy to see how, if you have more contact with multiple healthcare teams, you are more likely to experience harm in this way.

MDTs are now considered the norm in the NHS; this was not always the case. Willcocks (2018) noted that working in this way improves effectiveness, safety and team member well-being, while reducing clinical errors and hospitalisation. Changes focused on group dynamics and a leadership role within the team that moved to different members according to the need. Willcocks (2018, p. 4) notes, citing Bergman, that leaders can come to the fore in an organisation when *they are needed, when their relevant skills, knowledge and expertise are required by the team*, a collaborative view of leadership within a team or an organisation which allows for the existence of expertise in every member of the MDT. They acknowledge the challenges in linking with other organisations, such as primary care; you may have come across this in your placements, where the location you work at has limited outreach to other services. Although nurses have a huge role in that area, other allied health work takes place within that space, which can forge both formal and informal links. Willcocks (2018) suggests that the specialist nurses act as a 'boundary spanner' in creating and supporting links from the MDT to the other groups outside it. But they noted that different specialities may have different expectations, so that one speciality may have a culture of being led purely by medical teams and another may be used to moving leadership between members of the team, depending on the need of the moment.

Funding models impact this, with incentives encouraging competition rather than collaboration (Kotz and Dugdale, 2014), as do policies and procedures. The NHS Long Term Plan spoke about integrated care systems in learning disabilities and autism, and the expectation for reasonable adjustments (NHS England, 2019a). It is vital to understand the factors that may impact the ability of the team, including the person and their carers, to work together.

To do this, we need to plan on a much broader level: we need to consider commissioning and that means processes and pathways, and models of care. We know that having models of care, along with structured care processes and pathways, improves healthcare. These models have been defined as *a set of activities designed to assist patients and their support systems in managing medical conditions and related psychosocial problems more effectively, with the aim of improving patients' health status and reducing the need for medical services* (Bodenheimer and Berry-Millett, 2009, p. 2).

Care management tends to include the specific functions, goals, core tasks, the target population, differentiating features and the multi-level focus of the activity (Challis et al., 2018). But most of all, it requires authentic relationships between the patient, their support network and the staff (Kuluski et al., 2017). It should be based in the community, with primary care firmly involved (Karam et al., 2021).

Different models of care

Many models include elements such as evidence-based protocols and pathways, patient self-management and collaboration between professionals and systems. Most of them are community-based and relationship-focused, such as the chronic care model (see Figure 5.1) which is reflected throughout these other models (see Table 5.1).

Model	Elements
Stratified care	Targets according to patient characteristic
	Works within specialities
	Struggles with cross-boundary work
Care coordination	Organisation of patient care activities
	Relationship-focused
	Often community-focused
Complex care management	Interdisciplinary teams, involving care coordination and education
	Long-term work
	Support on accessing services or advocacy
	Relationship-focused

(Continued)

Table 5.1   (Continued)

Model	Elements
Hospital to home	Transition between systems
	Focus on early discharge and preventable readmissions
	Recovery from acute episodes
	Equipment, MDT support and care packages
Chronic disease self-management	Focused on specific conditions
	Interdisciplinary
	Relationship-focused
Chronic care model	Community recourses, healthcare organisation, self-management, delivery system design, decision support and clinical information
	(Figure 5.1)
Ask how I am	Continuity of care, information and partnership
	(Figure 5.2)

Table 5.1   Models of care (Mao et al., 2017; Reynolds et al., 2018)

Activity 5.1   Reflection

Think back to someone from your placement or your personal life and consider their experience of this type of model: can you think of many people who would benefit from this type of care?

As this activity is based on your own reflection, no outline answer is given at the end of this chapter.

All these models have existed in a variety of forms throughout the world's healthcare systems, with recurring elements. The role of the care coordinator is heavily used in complex needs, since the people living with those needs often have them long term and require similar support. The focus moves from health policy, supporting environments and community action, into the health system, exploring designs, self-management, decision support and information systems. The balance between the person living with complexity and a prepared proactive team is a key point, and one that you can see reflected in healthcare policy today. In this way, a person might move through levels of care within the team from intensive work as they are admitted, to step-down safety net support that can be withdrawn or stepped back up as needed.

The reality that patients experience may be different; Boehmer et al. (2018) suggested that the model does not consider the extra complexity and burden that living with multi-morbidity creates, which equally applies to living with complexity. Have a look at Figure 5.2 and consider how this model allows the person to exist as a holistic, complex being in comparison.

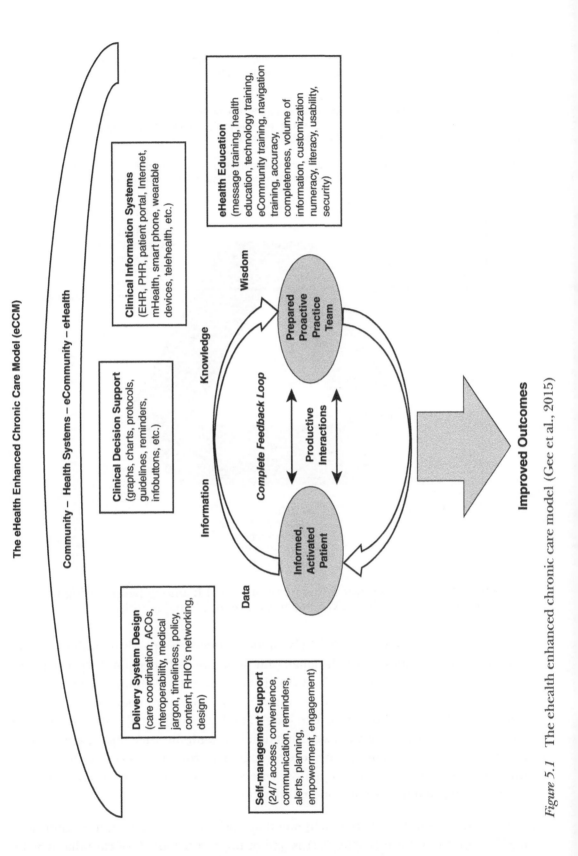

The eHealth Enhanced Chronic Care Model (eCCM)

Community – Health Systems – eCommunity – eHealth

eHealth Education
(message training, health education, technology training, eCommunity training, navigation training, accuracy, completeness, volume of information, customization numeracy, literacy, usability, security)

Clinical Information Systems
(EHR, PHR, patient portal, Internet, mHealth, smart phone, wearable devices, telehealth, etc.)

Clinical Decision Support
(graphs, charts, protocols, guidelines, reminders, infobuttons, etc.)

Delivery System Design
(care coordination, ACOs, Interoperability, medical jargon, timeliness, policy, content, RHIO's networking, design)

Self-management Support
(24/7 access, convenience, communication, reminders, alerts, planning, empowerment, engagement)

Wisdom

Knowledge

Information

Data

Complete Feedback Loop

Prepared Proactive Practice Team

Informed, Activated Patient

Productive Interactions

Improved Outcomes

Figure 5.1 The ehealth enhanced chronic care model (Gee et al., 2015)

Ask How I Am – a model of whole person care for people living with long-term physical health conditions

UNIVERSAL: continuity of care, information and partnership, routine enquiry about mental health, an annual holistic wellbeing check, and support for carers. These elements should be a feature of all long-term conditions services for everyone.

HOLISTIC: practical help (for example with money and work), mental health self-help resources, social prescribing and peer support. These should always be available freely when and where they are needed, offered proactively and equitably, adapted to people's needs and wishes.

SPECIALIST: a range of psychological therapies and interventions, mental health practitioners located within long-term conditions services and emotional support for carers. These should be 'on hand' to offer specialist support when it's required.

SPECIALIST
- Psychological therapies
- Collaborative care
- Mental health staff in long-term condition teams
- Carer mental health support

UNIVERSAL
- Continuity of care
- Annual wellbeing check
- Routine enquiry
- Carer support
- Information and partnership

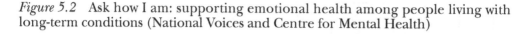

HOLISTIC
- Self-help resources
- Practical support
- Social prescribing
- Peer support

Figure 5.2   Ask how I am: supporting emotional health among people living with long-term conditions (National Voices and Centre for Mental Health)

One model, known as the Camden Core Model, targeted people living with complexities with frequent admissions to hospital, with no significant effect on the participants' readmission rate (Finkelstein et al., 2020). Therefore, it is important that quality trials are included in the evidence for these interventions, or we are asking our patients to expend effort to no or little avail. The King's Fund (Goodwin et al., 2013) recognised that the delivery of these services was often different, with the same objective to provide proactive approaches to bring care services together around the needs of the people living with complexity. There are many barriers to joint working, from individuals to commissioning and trans-organisational communication.

It does require a different approach, one that works from the person to commissioning. The House of Care (Figure 5.3) is one of the newer models of care that may be

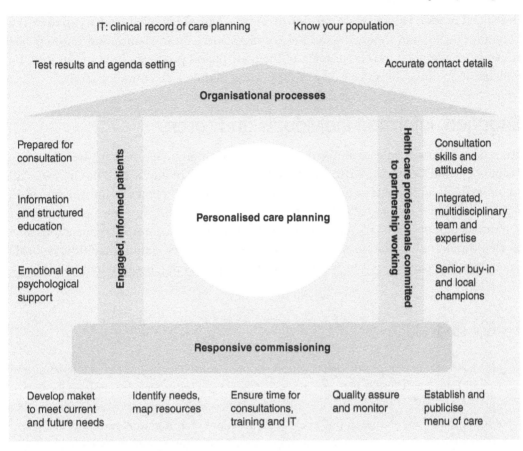

IT: clinical record of care planning   Know your population

Test results and agenda setting   Accurate contact details

Organisational processes

Prepared for consultation

Information and structured education

Emotional and psychological support

Engaged, informed patients

Personalised care planning

Helth care professionals committed to partnership working

Consultation skills and attitudes

Integrated, multidisciplinary team and expertise

Senior buy-in and local champions

Responsive commissioning

| Develop maket to meet current and future needs | Identify needs, map resources | Ensure time for consultations, training and IT | Quality assure and monitor | Establish and publicise menu of care |

Figure 5.3   House of Care (adapted from Coulter et al., 2016)

adapted for people living with complexity. Our original definition of complexity, it takes the point where the person meets the systems as the cause of the complexity, and this model works in that area.

House of Care

The House of Care framework was designed to create a coordinated service model for people with LTCs. It works equally well for people living with complexity – the support around them is intended to shape according to their needs (Coulter et al., 2016; Coulter et al., 2013). It was built on the chronic care model that we discussed earlier in the chapter, but with the NHS in mind. The aim is to embed the care planning and support for self-management into the system, and it contains several elements that we know are required for care to be collaborative on a systemic level.

Partnership working

Promoting and enhancing patient's motivation, knowledge, skills and confidence to manage their own conditions moves the healthcare team from the medical model into the social model, refocusing attention from the pathology of disease to an area that promotes health and well-being, and encourages and supports autonomy and self-care. It can be challenging to release some of the control and power we hold in our jobs, but collaboration and coherence is key in supporting people with complex needs.

Engaged, informed individuals and carers

We continue to struggle to support people in taking an active part in their own care (Chambers and Coleman, 2016). In the UK, 43 per cent of adults lack the literacy skills to understand food labels or instructions that come with medicines or information given out by the NHS. Enabling us to learn how we can support and trust our patients in their self-management is a challenge for all levels of health education. Organisations such as Healthwatch help people speak up and improve services, gaining confidence at the same time. You can see in John's experience the impact being involved had on his life.

Case study: John

John was referred to a psychologist for a series of 1:1 consultations to help him to learn to cope with his ME/CFS (at the time ME/CFS was considered to be a psychological condition). She identified that he had an underlying issue with uncompleted tasks and a sense of having a lack of a 'sense of purpose' – having retired early due to ill-health from a very interesting career. She set him a goal of decluttering his house over an extended period and to look for an interesting activity that he could cope with realistically. On completion of this decluttering, he felt improved mentally but still needed that sense of purpose. As a result, a little later he signed up as a volunteer with his local Healthwatch. He didn't get too many opportunities during the next two years due to a dip in his health but the one that 'turned him around' and gave him the sense of purpose was volunteering with a local university as an expert by experience on the nursing degree course. He had finally found that essential sense of purpose and is now involved at various levels with several health and care organisations (via Healthwatch in his county) including the university, NHS Hospitals Trust, the NHS Health and Care Trust and the NHS Clinical Commissioning Group plus quite a few others including voluntary and community sector (VCS) organisations. He has achieved the goal set by the psychologist!

Organisational and supporting processes

Creating models of care that allow for the necessary flexibility to meet these needs in a personalised way can be challenging. In service design, we set outcome measurements, intended to monitor the impact of our service on our intended target (Chapter 4).

Commissioning is vital for the House of Care to succeed, and measurement of success is part of the process. Clinical commissioning groups (CCGs) have measured amount of care plans and patient activation measurements (a self-reported measure to see if someone is ready to self-manage), alongside impacts such as individual admissions to hospital and use of healthcare services (Hart and Eastman, 2016). Various elements are required for the changes a CCG needs to make for House of Care to be successful:

- *ownership*: the change should belong to those working or living in that field or area, and so co-production is vital;
- *measurement*: completing the plan–do–study–act cycle is vital;
- *tailoring support to need*: ensure there is a baseline measurement because bringing in new IT systems (for example) would not succeed if staff or patients could not use them;
- *new skills*: motivational interviewing, goal-setting and coaching may be new to some staff members;
- *faith in the commitment for the long term*: the staff and patients need to believe that this is not something that will go away tomorrow and have the space and time to develop the skills and confidence they need to see the benefits;
- *good IT*: working templates and codes are vital to support this system. Patients being able to access their notes is a vital part of this;
- *contract and culture change*: the NHS is often incentivised by contracts and finances to deliver specific outcomes. Cultural changes are vital in turning the new way of working into the normal, routine business of the day.

(Hart and Eastman, 2016)

Commissioning including 'more than medicine'

At the foundation of the House of Care is the resources that exist in our community. Groups such as support groups, cookery classes, gardening projects, volunteer befriending are vital in this area. Social prescribing or community signposting relies on staff knowing what is available locally; see Chapter 10 to relate this to the care of a child and their family (Coulter et al., 2016). Local assets matter and doing the work around asset mapping is vital in knowing what your patients can access that might be right on their doorstep. In this case, an asset might be an organisation, a club, or a person.

Activity 5.2   Critical thinking

Look around your own local community – look online at the library and other locations that may have information – and make a list of the things your patients could access if they lived near you.

As this activity is based on your own thoughts, no outline answer is provided at the end of this chapter.

Scottish implementation

Greater Glasgow and Cylde NHS implemented and evaluated the House of Care (Leven, 2017). Although the patients did not know the name 'House of Care', they were aware that several elements had changed. Patients now received copies of their test results in writing before they went to the appointment with their healthcare professional. Some of them found that this motivated them to make changes:

> *I think as much as anything, you're going to take them more seriously because it reinforces them. It's easy to forget otherwise.*

(Leven, 2017, p.6)

In the same way, having their own written care plan was useful:

> *[The care plan] is a stark reminder. If it's out of sight, it's out of mind. If you go to the surgery they say to you, look this is what you need to do, and then you come away and that's it. But if you've got [the care plan] sitting there, then you have a look and you remember what you've got to do and why. So it's very helpful.*

(Leven, 2017, p.14)

Giving the patients time is important, and the feedback suggested that collaborative care was happening, including partners and family. The patients involved felt they were ready to self-manage, even if they occasionally struggled with willpower and perhaps didn't eat or exercise as they should. As you can see in Amara's case, having the test results or information in advance can be very empowering and allow the person to consider their options.

Case study: Amara

Amara, a cisgender woman with type 2 diabetes, depression and COPD, attended her information-gathering appointment and identified her COPD as her primary issue. She then received a copy of her test results and a care plan for her to fill out before her care planning conversation appointment. They had reviews with the practice nurse and the GP, with her partner in attendance.

These conversations allowed her to identify the limiting factors in her life (such as mobility), and she was supported to identify goals and monitor those goals with her own test results. During these conversations, issues around her weight and her mood were identified. She felt able to accept a referral to a weight management service and took home some information on a supportive service for her low mood.

Activity 5.3   Reflection

Review the above case study. What might be the barriers to this type of care? What benefits might Amara experience from this type of care?

A brief outline answer is provided at the end of this chapter.

Critiques of the House of Care model

The House of Care has very little mention of the residential sector; people with complex conditions may often reside in care homes, and much of the support that is directed towards the NHS for this work is lacking in that sector. While staff in the social care system are highly specialised professionals, they are often massively under-resourced and isolated from the NHS.

Another critique might include the difficulty in transitioning – either from one system to another, or from an aged service to another (child to adult, for example). It would need regular revisiting to make it useful for people who move between services in this way.

Let's look at transitional care, considering the impact of that movement between systems, services and locations on our person with complex care needs.

Transitional care

In all models of care, people move between systems, from hospital to home, or from paediatric systems to adult. For children, for example, they may be discharged back to their home after birth or hospital admissions with interventions that were previously hospital-based (Elias and Murphy, 2012). You may now see ventilators, intravenous catheters, tracheostomy tubes, feeding devices, colostomy bags and urinary catheters within the community, in adults and children alike (see Chapters 8 and 10). For this to succeed, the broad MDT must work together and first establish the place of care – although we acknowledge now that community and home is best, it is not always possible for all people. It relies on several elements, identified by Elias and Murphy (2012):

People. Is the person medically stable enough to be at home? Does the patient and the family want this to happen? Have they got the necessary skills, resources (time, energy, finances) to do this?

Home. Is the home adequate, safe, and accessible? Does it have more than the basics – some conditions may require air conditioning in some climates, for example. A back-up generator for a ventilator would be wise.

Community: Who is available to support them at home? This may be the community healthcare team including the GP, practice nurses and district nurses, their specialist team, pharmacist, support groups and emergency services. Some people, including children and people with learning disabilities, may have lifelong need for nursing care, and this may be endangered by the shortage of nurses.

Training: There needs to be a movement from the hospital doing the care, to training those involved (family or paid carers), including a supportive transition.

School and education: For children or young people who are still going through education, it should be considered how they will access this. They may need additional support, both in terms of accessibility and support.

In some countries, much of this relies on the insurance and financial situation of the family. Someone with good insurance or a solid financial position may be able to afford to supply these things, while someone who is not in such a good position may struggle to access them. In the UK, we are lucky in that we have the NHS and the social care system, both of which should meet most of these needs.

Good transitional care in paediatrics includes several components:

- Patient engagement:
  - goal-setting
  - patients as partners
  - monitoring progress towards goals
  - enabling communication
  - continuity of care.
- Caregiver engagement:
  - comprehensive assessments with caregivers as partners
  - monitoring progress towards goals
  - enabling communication.
- Complexity and medication management:
  - identification of high-risk patients
  - anticipatory planning for common problems
  - managing risks
  - preventing post-hospital syndrome
  - aligning services with goals
  - medication management plan based on evidence
  - respecting patient choice in concordance with plan
  - access to medications.
- Patient education:
  - identifying health literacy and language level
  - accessible, accurate health information
  - confirmation of understanding of information/instructions.

- Caregiver education:
  - involvement in planning care
  - respecting and valuing their contributions
  - provision of information and training
  - support.
- Patients' and caregivers' well-being:
  - early identification and interventions to address emotional distress
  - recognition of common concerns and reactions to their role
  - identification and implementation of strategies to support their emotional well-being.
- Care continuity:
  - ensuring follow-up with appropriate services
  - communicating effectively between teams
  - encouraging respectful, reciprocal relationships built on trust
  - accountability
  - fulfilling responsibilities in a comprehensive and timely manner
  - collaborating as a team to make sure goals and preferences are met.

(Naylor et al., 2017)

As you can see, the complexities of moving from one location or service to another does allow for errors to occur. In the scenario below, you can see the opportunities for the transitional care to be good or poorly completed.

Case study: going home

Marie, a 25-year-old cisgender woman, had her baby four weeks prematurely and had to spend time in the neonatal intensive care unit. The staff there have been preparing the family to go home with enough skills and support to continue their journey. The preparation included training in the care of their baby and learning skills to look after them without harming the very delicate body (see Chapter 10 for more on this).

Activity 5.4   Reflection

Thinking about your own lives, consider what support you might need to go home in similar circumstances? Who might you need to support you?

As this activity is based on your own reflection, no outline answer is given at the end of this chapter.

The transition from child to adult services can be equally problematic here; the NICE guideline for ADHD defines the transition as a referral to the adult service being made and accepted, the first appointment attended (see Chapter 10 for more on transitional care). Optimum transition should include joint care, planning meetings, information transfer and continuity of care (Eke et al., 2020). In ADHD in particular, Eke et al. (2020) found that there was a low rate of successful transition and those guidelines were not followed well. It is considered a dangerous time for some people living with complexity, where the conflict between independence and dependency causes young people to feel lacking in control (Dallimore et al., 2018). This may be between the young person and their family, as control moves between them. This situation requires delicate management from the care team to support the family in letting the young person find their feet in managing their own condition.

Case study: helping Harry make choices

As a child with complex care needs, Harry often needed to have painful and frightening treatments for his haemophilia and had no control over when he needed them. They often occurred at times of injury (aka bleeds into joints), which were painful and required unplanned trips to hospital.

To allow Harry control over some aspects of his care, Harry's parents, Rosemary and Eddie, ensured that he was in control of who gave his treatments, the location of them and who was around him. In giving him the right to control this and make the limited choices available, he felt more able to engage with the treatment. They were careful to ensure that these hospital trips were linked with fun treats for both Harry and Hermione, his sister.

The young person may feel they lack information on how to navigate the new systems; what happens if they go to university or move house? That information may come from new sources, such as forums, social media, or support groups, and may be of variable quality – we'll explore this in more detail shortly!

Activity 5.5   Reflection

Before you read on, think about where you get information for your own healthcare needs. Make a list and consider how reliable those sources are. Do your friends, outside healthcare, use the same or different sources?

As this activity is based on your own reflection, no outline answer is given at the end of this chapter.

Information sources

Despite the assumption that young people may not be able to identify poor sources of information, Freeman et al. (2018) demonstrated that they were well equipped to assess web sources and are keenly aware of the varying quality of online information. Hausmann et al. (2017) found that 99 per cent of young people use social media and half of them had shared health information there. The majority of that related to mood, wellness or a specific medical condition and they were more likely to share if they had poor health. They demonstrated that young people do not view social media as a useful source of health information.

Parents do use the internet as a default information source about their child's treatment but tended to consult with healthcare professionals as well. But Benedicta et al. (2020) found that their abilities to find, understand and appraise that information were not strong. It is important that healthcare professionals provide information and link parents and patients to resources that are reliable, comprehensive and easy to understand. Although sometimes these conversations can be challenging, depending on the topic, it is vital that we have them (Schmidt et al., 2021).

In general, supporting people with the knowledge they need to find information and identify good sources is a key part of self-management, but sometimes people take control and become very active, both in their care and in creating changes in society. These are known as health social movements.

Health social movements

Throughout this chapter we have spoken about what we, as healthcare professionals, can and should be doing; we as people equally have some responsibility to take control and drive changes in our system. Mathers and Paynton (2016) noted that patients need to be active participants in their care, and more broadly that patients can start health social movements. You will be familiar with at least one of these: Kate Granger's '*Hello, my name is…*' movement. These have been around for as long as healthcare has, ranging from expansion of reproductive rights to altered treatment forms in breast cancer (Brown et al., 2004). Campaigns against stigma and for disability rights are part of this movement, and we can align ourselves alongside our patients, lifting their stories into visibility and using the power of our positions to support them in their own movements.

Chapter summary

In this chapter, we have discussed the MDTs and their role in bringing care together. We have talked about the House of Care, and we have discussed how commissioning could be

(Continued)

(Continued)

a part of that. Remember in Chapter 2 we discussed integrated care systems, and hopefully now you can link those partnerships between organisations to the House of Care and other chronic disease management models of care.

Each of the approaches we have discussed have certain characteristics in common; most had MDT care, comprehensive assessment and case management. They found that training and decision support were key factors, and integration across teams, organisations and systems were useful.

But at the centre of all of them was the patient and their needs. In the next chapter, we'll discuss assessment processes that can place the patient at the heart and attempts to avoid having to repeat their story to a dozen different healthcare professionals.

Activities: brief outline answers

Activity 5.3 Reflection (page 73)

Time is a major barrier – a GP appointment is often seven minutes, and practice nurses experience a similar pressure on their time. As skilled professionals, the practice nurses can complete their specialist assessment in that time, but it reduces the chances of identifying the secondary issues. The preparation work before the appointment requires time and joined up teamwork – the GP and practice nurses are not the only team members in the surgery, and this brings in the administration staff, who often work behind the scenes to keep the wheels running.

The benefits far outweigh the challenges: Amara would have had time to digest and explore the information she was given, instead of having to do so in an appointment. She would have had time to discuss it with her partner and the time and space to discuss her options.

Annotated further reading

Stárek, L. (2021) The base and development of multidisciplinary collaboration. *Psychology and Education Journal,* 58(5), 3017–21.

This article provides an insight into multidisciplinary management in psychology.

Karam, M., et al. (2021) Nursing care coordination for patients with complex needs in primary healthcare: a scoping review. *International Journal of Integrated Care,* 21(1), 16.

This article explores care coordination and will give you some insight into that area of practice.

Useful websites

https://www.england.nhs.uk/ourwork/clinical-policy/ltc/house-of-care/

This page is the home for the House of Care and includes a lot of useful resources.

https://www.yearofcare.co.uk/year-care-solution

This page explores the House of Care further.

Chapter 6 Shared decision-making

NMC Future Nurse: Standards of Proficiency for Registered Nurses

This chapter will address the following platforms and proficiencies:

Platform 1: Being an accountable professional

1.9 understand the need to base all decisions regarding care and interventions on people's needs and preferences, recognising and addressing any personal and external factors that may unduly influence their decisions

1.14 provide and promote non-discriminatory, person-centred and sensitive care at all times, reflecting on people's values and beliefs, diverse backgrounds, cultural characteristics, language requirements, needs and preferences, taking account of any need for adjustments

Platform 3: Assessing needs and planning care

3.6 effectively assess a person's capacity to make decisions about their own care and to give or withhold consent

3.8 understand and apply the relevant laws about mental capacity for the country in which you are practising when making decisions in relation to people who do not have capacity

Platform 4: Providing and evaluating care

4.2 work in partnership with people to encourage shared decision-making in order to support individuals, their families and carers to manage their own care when appropriate

> ## Chapter aims
>
> After reading this chapter, you will be able to:
>
> - critique the process of shared decision-making, and who should be involved in the process to aid effective and efficient solutions and the polices which serve to enable it
> - assess the roles of the professional team in enabling patient choice in decision-making and distinguish between information that is relevant to care planning and information that is not
> - detect the barriers to shared decision-making in the adult, child and young person and discuss what, if anything, can be done to overcome them
> - predict ethical considerations which may arise in the process of shared decision-making.

Introduction

In this chapter, we'll be looking at how we make decisions with the people living with complex needs; often decisions are made about them, rather than with them. Sometimes this is about process and speed of decision-making, but other times it may be about the clinician's skill level in communicating with someone who may have challenges in that area. There are some legal issues around capacity to consider.

What is shared decision-making?

Shared decision-making (SDM) is a key part of person-centred care in every field of nursing (Waldron et al., 2020). We sit with our patients together to reach an agreement on tests or treatments. It is vital to bring information and evidence into that discussion with the person, together with their values and preferences to come to a decision – think of evidence-based practice with the best evidence, choice, preferences and ethics, alongside the clinician's knowledge. It allows evidence and choice to become part of the evidence-based practice we all aim to provide. This sounds so obvious, but only 39 per cent of patients felt they were involved in SDM during their appointments and 37 per cent wanted to be more involved than they were (Waldron et al., 2020). Sadly, a survey by the Nuffield Trust showed that this had not changed much over time at all (Nuffield Trust, 2021).

When people are well informed, they make different choices about their treatment, and those decisions are often different to those their clinicians were expecting (Mulley et al., 2012). For people whose identity is being eroded, from social position changes or disease progression, upholding their personhood is vital and something that nurses are particularly skilled at. Acknowledgement of the person as a partner in their own care and decisions improves quality of care (and may reduce costs since not everyone wants to be treated when we assume they would!). Additionally, one of the reasons we need to pause in these decisions is that we often do not have an accurate perception of the risks or benefits of a chosen treatment, often minimising the harms and overstating the benefits (Hoffmann and Del Mar, 2017).

Activity 6.1   Reflection

Pause for a moment and write a brief person-centred care plan for yourself: what would you need in it, if you knew you were going to experience memory loss or cognitive changes tomorrow, to uphold your own personhood?

As this activity is based on your own reflection, no outline answer is given at the end of this chapter.

When we start with keeping our patients in our minds as people with their own rights, preferences and ethics, shared decision-making (SDM) is an obvious choice. After all, imagine if someone else got to decide what you wear, eat and do all day? But we assume that we can make those choices for some of our patients who may have cognitive or communication issues. For people with complex needs, this SDM is vital, since their most pressing issue may not be the one that you would prioritise. SDM moves from the paternalistic model and acts as a balance between clinician and the patient. When we provide healthcare, we aim for quality: safe, effective, person-centred, timely, equitable and efficient. The Health Foundation (2012) used the following definition:

> *Shared decision-making is a process in which clinicians and patients work together to select tests, treatments, management, or support packages, based on clinical evidence and the patient's informed preferences. It involves the provision of evidence-based information about options, outcomes, and uncertainties, together with decision support counselling and a system for recording and implementing patients' informed preferences.*

(p. 2)

It is worth noting that, while they are connected concepts, self-management and SDM are different things (Health Foundation, 2014b). SDM places emphasis on information to make a decision or take an action around their health, whereas self-management supports people to bring that evidence into their lives and make changes to manage their day-to-day lives. Similarly, you should be able to spot the links to person-centred care (PCC), where both SDM and PCC put these principles at the centre:

- affording people dignity, compassion and respect;
- coordinated care, support, or treatment;
- personalised care, support, or treatment;
- enabling people to build their own capabilities.

If we start from an ethical viewpoint that it is just the right thing to do with our patients, what does that look like in practice? In practice we use a variety of models; here are three for you to explore.

Models of SDM in practice

There are the following key themes in the majority of SDM models:

- make the decision
- patient preferences
- tailor information
- deliberate
- create choice awareness
- learn about the patient.

(Bomhof-Roordink et al., 2019)

This included time outside the face-to-face consultations, giving the patient time in their own world to consider the information, find more or speak with others (remember the information sources from Chapter 5). But three models provide further structure for us to use in our practice which we will now explore in more detail:

- three-talk model of SDM
- interprofessional SDM model
- Ottawa Decision Support Framework.

Three-talk model of SDM

During the process of sharing information, active listening is a key communication skill since it could become a tick-box exercise. It is worthy of note that this model contains only one clinician and the patient. But in complex care nursing, we operate in MDTs (see Chapter 5), and there may be a particular team member who is acting as the lead in that case, or more than one person who should be in the room with the patient (be that another professional involved in their care or an advocate, carer, or family member).

Elwyn et al. (2017) suggested this model of SDM brings together evidence-based practice and person-centred care and outlined the three stages in the three-talk model. Later, Elwyn and Vermunt (2020) included the visualisation tool called a goal board, adding the word 'goal' to each of the three stages, asking patient and clinician to prioritise a goal in the Team Talk stage, consider the impact on the goal at the Option Talk stage (changing the priority if necessary) and making the decisions based on the goals with a plan to evaluate it at the Decision Talk stage (Figure 6.1). Example questions that the clinician might use include 'what activities do you want to be able to carry on doing?', or 'what symptom or aspect of disease do you want to change?'. The goals can

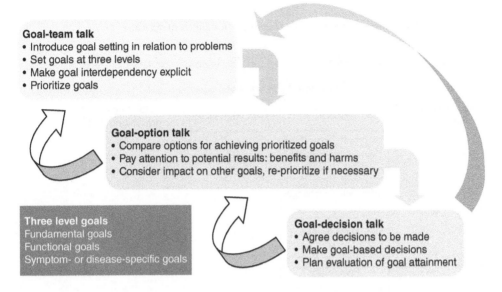

Goal-team talk
- Introduce goal setting in relation to problems
- Set goals at three levels
- Make goal interdependency explicit
- Prioritize goals

Goal-option talk
- Compare options for achieving prioritized goals
- Pay attention to potential results: benefits and harms
- Consider impact on other goals, re-prioritize if necessary

Three level goals
Fundamental goals
Functional goals
Symptom- or disease-specific goals

Goal-decision talk
- Agree decisions to be made
- Make goal-based decisions
- Plan evaluation of goal attainment

Figure 6.1 Goal-based shared decision-making model (Elwyn and Vermunt, 2020)

then be set onto a visual board, into high, medium and low priorities. Decision aids are useful and we'll talk about them in more depth later in this chapter.

Interprofessional SDM model

This model is broader than the three-talk model, considering those people we mentioned before. It gives more space for the process to be less linear in nature; there is a natural back and forth in these decisions where information is clarified and preferences identified. The aim is a much more person-centred decision, and it fits the MDT working for complex care nursing much better.

It includes three levels in the healthcare system: the micro (individual) level, the meso (healthcare teams in an organisation) level and the macro (social context and policies) level. The complex care team may sit within the meso level of this, acting as a decision coach.

It includes those outside the person themselves and their current healthcare professional. There are two axes – the vertical one shows the decision moving through time, interacting with the need to consider values, how viable the options are and so on (Figure 6.2). The other axis contains those who may be involved, and therefore shows the movement between different people.

Ottawa Decision Support Framework

This model seeks to use decision aids to improve the SDMs, using these tools to prepare both clinicians and patients for the conversation and decision. It provides certain parts of SDM that should be in place for quality decisions to be made.

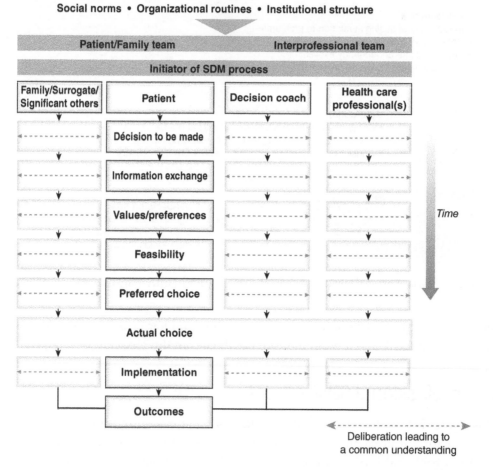

Figure 6.2 The IP-SDM model (Légaré et al., 2014 under Creative Commons Attribution License 4.0)

You can see that Figure 6.3 shows the intersection of the resources needed for a decision to be made by the patient, their supporters and the healthcare team. It considers the decision's own properties such as urgency, taking the available support for that (such as decision aids, motivational interviewing, etc.) and linking them to the improvement of outcome we are seeking, aka the quality of the decision-making process.

Patient activation and preparation

One of the things we know is that for SDM we need all partners to be active in that decision and be willing to take that active role, to feel confident and either have, or be willing to learn, the skills to manage their care and make those choices. The MAGIC programme is a good example of using campaigns to activate people in their own care, including patients as stakeholders in the design process. Another example of this type of campaign is the Ask Share Know campaign, which showed similar benefits.

Decisional Needs
- Difficult decision type/timing
- Unreceptive decisional stage
- Decisional conflict (uncertainty)
- Inadequate knowledge & unrealistic expectations
- Unclear values
- Inadequate support & resources*
- Personal & clinical needs

Decisional Outcomes
Quality of the decision
- Informed
- Values-based

Quality of the decision making process
- Reduced decisional needs

Impact
- Implementation continuance of chosen option
- Appropriate use & costs of health services

Decision Support
- **Establish rapport & facilitate interactive communication**
- **Clarify decision & invite participation**
- **Assess decisional needs**
- **Address decisional needs with tailored support:**
  - Facilitate receptivity to information/deliberation
  - Provide information/outcome probabilities & verify understanding
  - Clarify personal values: option features that matter most
  - Discuss decisional roles
  - Support deliberation & mobilize resources
  - Monitor decisional needs &/ facilitate progress in decisional making stages

Clinical Counseling	**Decision Tools**	**Decision Coaching**

Figure 6.3　Ottawa Decision Support Framework (replicated with the kind permission of University of Ottawa)

These campaigns tend to only appear in a waiting room. Most healthcare for complex needs takes place in a person's home and so that is rather late to change ideas, beliefs, or attitudes (Joseph-Williams et al., 2014a). Leaflets or information before the appointment allow the person to consider their options, list their questions and discuss them with their support network. Some of that preparation can involve the use of decision aids.

Shared decision aids

The three-talk model and the Ottawa Decision Support Framework are, as we said, designed for specific treatments or tests and are collected into the International Patient Decision Aid Standards Collaboration. For example, you might find some around cervical cancer screening, childbirth options, or fibroid treatment. They are provided in a range of formats to allow patients to use the communication best suited to them – so you could pick from pamphlets, videos, or websites to help people to understand their options from their own point of view.

Activity 6.2   Reflection

Considering your last placement, go to the IPDASC and see if you can find a relevant decision aid.

- What resources are available for the condition or treatment you have in mind?
- Would you find it useful?
- Critique the decision aid of your choice. What are the strengths and weaknesses?

As this activity is based on your own reflection, no outline answer is given at the end of this chapter.

Stacey et al. (2017) found that using these made patients feel more informed and knowledgeable about their options; they generally took a greater role in making their decisions, understanding the risks they may face.

Taking this further, although websites and leaflets are useful outside the appointment, Joseph-Williams et al. (2017) found that brief decision aids were much better at helping the conversation along. They found that it encouraged patients to ask the questions and discuss what was important to them but that any tool can be used as a tick-box exercise. In the scenario below, Geoff was able to take advantage of the time he had to consider his options and the GP spent time with him to discuss those within the appointment.

Case study: SDM consultation

After discovering that his blood pressure was too high, Geoff scheduled a GP appointment to discuss it. Before going, his GP provided him with a written decision aid, with information about his options, by post (you can see it at this website: https://www.nice.org.uk/guidance/ng136/resources/how-do-i-control-my-blood-pressure-lifestyle-options-and-choice-of-medicines-patient-decision-aid-pdf-6899918221).

This gave Geoff some time to consider his options and do more research, talking to a friend who is a nurse and reading some information online from various sources. He was able to come to the appointment with a list of questions and a preference that would suit him – to first try lifestyle changes. His GP spent time talking through the options with him (bringing together the three parts of evidence-based practice). The consultation ended with the GP referring Geoff to an 'exercise by prescription' scheme to help him.

You can see from the scenario how a decision aid might help us to walk through the conversation, both providing the information about the options and giving the patient the space they need to speak up.

What about if the evidence is unclear?

Understanding the context in which your patient is making a decision can be key in aiding the clinician in situations where the decision is less clear, or less well supported by literature and evidence. This can often be the case for people with complex care needs – for example, when pain management medication may have an adverse effect on the kidney function, but without that, the person's quality of life is poor. It is important to remember that these things might be conditional or change over time; if the pain is at the level where the person can cope, then they might prioritise the kidney function, but if the symptoms worsen, that may change. Equally, if it is a side-effect of the medication (constipation for example), being aware of that context might mean you could offer an alternative. The other context you may need to consider includes the legal and ethical context of the decision being made.

Legalities

Whatever the context of the decision itself, you need to be mindful of several legal frameworks, including the Mental Capacity Act (Department of Health, 2005) and the Children's Act (Perera, 2008) – you will find more on all of these in Chapters 9 and 10. Broadly, we need to make sure our process of consent is clear and fits within the definition provided by the Mental Health Act Commission:

> *[for] consent to be effective, [it] must be a 'real' consent. It must be genuine, uninfluenced by coercion or by fraud or misdescription, and it must be based on sufficient information.*

> (Mental Health Act Commission, 1985, p. 3, cited by Thomas and Forbes (1989, p. 4))

The law now requires us to take *reasonable care to ensure that the patient is aware of any material risks involved in any recommended treatment, and of any reasonable alternative or variant treatments* (Montgomery v Lanarkshire, 2015, p. 29).

This means that we, as clinicians, are legally bound to provide our patients with the ability to make a true decision and provide true consent. In complex care nursing, we find the increased need for them to be observed and implemented. If you are making a decision with someone with capacity, with a single condition and no other challenges that may be included in the complex needs area, this can be comparatively straightforward. This changes when there are more issues and challenges, many of which we find in the lives of those living with complex needs.

Capacity

Shared decision-making may require a capacity assessment (see Chapters 7 and 10). Guidry-Grimes (2020) notes this as one of the challenges in SDM in the mental health field.

If they do not have the legal capacity to consent to treatment or to make a decision, then best interest actions may be required. This would fall under the frameworks of the Mental Capacity Act Code of Practice (Department for Constitutional Affairs, 2005) and the NICE guidelines of decision-making and mental capacity (National Institute for Health and Care Excellence, see Annotated further reading). We'll discuss this more in Chapters 7, 9 and 10.

Different populations

When we consider SDM, we need to be aware of the different needs and methods within different populations and groups of people – after all, many of those with complex needs fall into those groups. For some, it might be around abilities and different forms of communication and, for others, we may need to consider the legalities of the situation. Remember that competency depends on the decision being made and the capacity of the person being able to make it.

Young people

When treating young people, the power imbalance is broader and their ability to engage in SDM varies by age, at the very least. The Children Act 1989, Section 105, defined a child as someone under eighteen (Young, 2019). To understand SDM in children and young people, you should be aware of Gillick competency and Fraser guidelines (more in Chapter 10) (NSPCC, 2020).

Coyne et al. (2014) defined SDM as *the ways in which children can contribute to the decision-making process, independent of who makes the final decision* (p. 274). Not involving them heightens their fear and anxiety, reduces their self-esteem and leaves them unprepared for the procedures they will experience. Lin et al. (2018) noted that for children with complex needs, including asthma, attention deficit hyperactivity disorder and type 1 diabetes, SDM was linked to decreased disease severity. They found that the reverse was true for where low SDM was occurring – those families had increased disability and higher costs.

But children and young people's ability to engage in SDM is often limited by life-threatening diagnosis, the urgency and the seriousness of their conditions. Coyne et al. (2014) provided context for this, stating that parents viewed their role as giving permission rather than making decisions, basing their choice on the trust they placed in the clinicians. We may see change as children grow and want an increased role and control over their own body, responding to the limitations placed on their autonomy with frustration, non-adherence to treatment and feelings of inadequacy and anger (Wicks and Mitchell, 2010). There might be smaller issues such as who is present or doing the treatment, such as those discussed in the Harry scenario.

Case study: Harry

Harry required a regular home treatment to prevent his bleeds. It was painful and could be scary since it was delivered through his implanted port in his chest. Although he had been involved in the decision to have this implanted, he found the process of the treatments difficult, particularly due to bad experiences with needles in the past.

To ensure that Harry had control over his body and decisions, as far as possible, he was firmly in charge of who delivered the treatment and who was allowed to be in the room.

Mental health

SDM in mental health practice comes with challenges that may not exist in other areas: the focus therefore is often on different outcomes, rather than decisions of care (Zisman-Ilani et al., 2021) (see Chapter 7 for an in-depth discussion on capacity). Measured outcomes for SDM in mental health might include empowerment, self-determination and recovery, many of which are rather difficult to measure objectively with validated tools (Zisman-Ilani et al., 2021). There can be an assumption on patients' (in)ability to be involved, but people with mental health challenges do desire to be and can be engaged in SDM (Alsulamy et al., 2020). In the Changing Relationships project, they provided training, materials and support to staff to begin to engage young people in SDM, but found that, while it had a good impact, there were some interesting findings (Health Foundation, 2014a). People needed to have time to be in the right space for them to engage with the SDM – there may be a crisis that needs resolving before that is possible, and some young people needed support to help them understand what was being asked of them. Aoki (2020) found that the relationship between the clinician and the patient, the communication process, user-friendly visualisation and stakeholder inclusion were key in SDM for mental health. Communication was certainly the most important of these and may be able to override the power issues inherent in mental health decision-making (Aoki, 2020).

Decision aids in psychiatry are rooted in evidence-based practice but are developed in a medical model focused on diagnosis which may not account for the complexity of psychiatric conditions (see Chapter 7 for much more on this). But one thing the Changing Relationships project discovered was that the tools do not ensure that SDM has taken place; there needs to be an individual and cultural shift to change the underpinning relationships with their patients. If it becomes a tick-box exercise, it really won't help your patients and may just become another piece of paperwork to fill in. Zisman-Ilani et al. (2021) challenge the NICE guidelines for SDM, stating that they do not address the differences that mental health requires, nor do they consider anything but a Western culture. Again, you can see the importance of understanding intersectionality in care.

We might find a variety of clinical tools that we can use to assess capacity, such as the mini-mental status examination, but often these just feed into a broader picture of the situation the person is in. It is vital that the clinician and the team involved in this document all the details that have bought them to the decision that the person does not have capacity to consent or make a decision. Once that decision has been made, there are several options; the questions the team might ask include the urgency of the choice – can this be delayed until the person has capacity or not (you can read more about capacity in Chapter 7)? The other primary question is whether they have a legal representative that might allow them to have a choice through a surrogate.

Case study: Harold

Harold has had a neurodegenerative condition for the last five years and is staying at a care home for respite. He has become more confused, hallucinating overnight and demanding to go home. He seems to think he is in the army barracks, where he used to work twenty years ago.

The care home calls the GP, who tests for a urine infection and starts antibiotics.

Activity 6.3   Reflection

If you were the care home nurse, what capacity assessments might you consider? Does he have the capacity to decide to go home? What activities could you use to help him navigate those experiences right now?

As this activity is based on your own reflection, no outline answer is given at the end of this chapter.

Learning disabilities

Learning disabilities (LD) is another area where there are challenges faced for SDM (see Chapter 9). Golnik et al. (2012) found that, where there was SDM, families reported more satisfaction and better guidance for treatments for children with autism spectrum disorders. There is still much work to be done. In general, the process in learning disabilities will bring professionals together with the person themselves and their family – as well as close supporters the person wants involved – to come to an agreement on the best course of action and best interests (you can read more about this in Chapter 9) (Royal College of Nursing, 2012). We should be ensuring that people with learning disabilities have opportunities to make choices as an equal partner in their care. The Department of Health guidance on consent for professionals working with people with learning disabilities may be a useful document for you to explore.

Campaigns by those affected by poor practices and lacking SDM in health, such as Oliver's Campaign, have worked to highlight the importance and urgency of this, resulting in changes such as the introduction of training across the NHS (Oliver's Campaign, n.d.).

Case study: Maria

Maria is 33 years old and has Down's syndrome; she lives in a community home with five others with learning disabilities.

Maria is generally in good health, is mobile and can use the toilet independently (with reminders to go), but needs help with other daily activities.

She is verbal and uses sentences with up to two key words, i.e.

- 'Maria go in *car* to the *shops*'
- 'Maria go *swimming* with *Brenda* (her friend)'
- '*Doggy* goes *Woof!*'

It is generally thought that her receptive language (what she understands) is better than her spoken; she can understand sentences like:

- 'Maria, will you go *upstairs* and get your *coat* to go to *church*'

Maria does not read, but is able to understand what is going on in pictures in a magazine, comic, story book or even on television. You can use pictures with her to ask questions and plan things – for example, you might see a seaside picture in a magazine and ask her if she likes the seaside or wants to go there, and she will answer correctly.

Maria understands simple symbols and drawn representations of things (dog, toilet, car, etc), and recognises pictures of places she knows, such as 'Church', 'Shops', 'Mummy's House'.

Maria likes and plays with dolls and likes to 'look after' and care for them, copying from other people (staff, family, TV, etc.). If she is watching a TV show where someone cuddles someone, she will copy by cuddling her doll.

Maria likes Mary, who lives with her, and likes to do things with Mary (who is a little older), seeing her as a role model; she copies what she does. Mary acts as an affectionate, respected 'big sister' to Maria.

Maria has an excellent relationship with her key worker Julia and will often engage in activities with Julia that she won't for other people.

Maria spends time with her parents; her father is particularly a trusted authority figure.

(Continued)

(Continued)

Maria has contact with Jenny, a community Learning Disabilities Nurse (who has supported the team with some minor behaviour issues before); she has had an excellent trusting relationship with Maria since she was a little girl.

Maria has always been anxious about going to doctors/dentist, etc., but used to tolerate having injections; recently she has developed a needle phobia, following a bad experience at their surgery with a practice nurse who could not find a vein, bruising her arm badly.

Activity 6.4   Reflection

What challenges might Maria face with healthcare? Reflect on your placements and how you might make reasonable adjustment there.

As this activity is based on your own reflection, no outline answer is given at the end of this chapter.

Barriers to SDM

Since it is such an obvious and simple concept, it would make sense for us to see this everywhere. After all, SDM was introduced in 1980, which is now more than 40 years ago. Waldron et al. cited literature which found several things that might stop physicians from using SDM in their practice, even when they are trying to do so (Shepherd et al. and Joseph-Williams et al., cited in Waldron et al., 2020). We will now explore some common barriers to SDM.

We already do it

Most clinicians already believe they do SDM with their patients. But the figures earlier in the chapter suggest that the patients do not entirely agree with that. Skills training helped narrow this gap; role play worked best in this situation, moving those involved from certainty that they were already doing this, to a willingness to improve their skills and practice in this area (Joseph-Williams et al., 2017).

We lack the right tools

Although there are many different decision aid tools, Joseph-Williams et al. (2017) found that when they trained clinicians, their skills and – more importantly – attitude changes meant much more than the use of the correct decision-making aid. It was clear that if they return to a team where this is not the norm, they will lapse back into their previous behaviour (Health Foundation, 2014b). It therefore requires an entire cultural change within the teams.

How can we measure it?

This is an issue since we do want to know what difference it makes in our practice and for our patients. Any PROMs may be biased due to the patient wanting to give us high satisfaction rating or their own knowledge on SDM and what it should look like.

Too many competing demands and priorities

Brogan et al. (2018) found that the clinicians involved were not sure what SDM was, who should start it, who should be involved and how to do it. The clinicians would engage in SDM conversations when the patient initiated it but specialist nurses engaged in watchful waiting, using the emerging new symptoms as a trigger event to start conversations about the future. Organisational factors were part of this. The specialist team felt that it was the role of the GP, whereas the GPs said that they were facilitators for the specialist nurses to lead that conversation. Alongside the case-load pressures and silo working this has created a space where SDM is fragmented and often late and task-focused. The recent crisis and pressures in the health and social care sector means that the communication becomes a casualty, with people fighting fire.

Would you want speedy treatment or time to think about your decision? If we incentivise the former, the latter may become less of an option for a patient to whom this a priority. Outcome measurements becomes targets: when leadership demonstrated a commitment to SDM as a quality issue and valued clinicians led and implemented it, it became a 'business as usual' issue rather than yet another initiative or poster on the wall. But the clinicians need clarity about whose role it is, and support with implementation such as lengthening appointment times (requiring more investment in staff) (Alsulamy et al., 2020).

Some of this may be due to implementation of SDM and changes to policies without changing the systems and organisations we have, which made it harder for clinicians to do this work. Others have raised concerns about unintended consequences; they suggested that when policy incentivised SDM it has it turned it into another check-box, particularly in areas where it is not a single decision. For example, Blumenthal-Barby et al. (2019) identified long-term conditions and complex needs as areas where it needs to be an ongoing rather than a single conversation. They noted that the early SDM models were (as we discussed earlier in this chapter) only focused on involving the patient.

Patients don't want it

The evidence shows that patients do want it, but at different levels or they fear the consequences of demanding it. Some older patients have been trained in the paternalistic model of care, or others may fear annoying the clinician (Alsulamy et al., 2020).

We might conceive of collaborations that can be different from this recommendation model, moving from a risk of the patient being perceived as 'good' if they accept that recommendation towards autonomy, including their social and cultural viewpoint and preferences (Elwyn et al., 2016). Relationship power imbalances change where SDM happens, since knowledge is not sufficient without the power (Joseph-Williams et al., 2014b). Simple measures (posters in the waiting rooms) can influence the person's self-efficacy by providing them with tools in the form of questions ('What are my options?', 'What are the benefits and harms?', 'How likely are these?'). Passive assent is not SDM.

Brogan et al. (2018) noted that patients are allowed to delegate the decision to others such as their clinicians – not doing something or only doing parts of it is a perfectly valid decision to make. Some SDM tools (such as SDM-Q-9) score the patient on how much they want to be involved in their decisions, scoring them low on their ability or willingness to engage. But despite that score, it is important to remember that they have engaged; they have decided that they want the decision to be made by a clinician. This is a perfectly reasonable choice; this patient may, for example, want to know the information but leave the decision itself to the clinician, as we can see in the case of Georgia.

Case study: Georgia

Harriet, a specialist nurse in neurology, received a referral for Georgia, a 60-year-old lady with multiple systems atrophy. Part of the care provided by the specialist nurses was to engage in the advance care planning for a rapidly progressing condition which would impact on Georgia's ability to communicate. When this topic was raised, Georgia was clear that she did not want to receive education on her condition or make advance plans, but to address each as they arose.

Activity 6.5   Critical thinking

Considering the case study above, what approach should Harriet take now to Georgia's care? Assess the ways in which she can balance the need to provide advance care planning and SDM without breaching the ethical imperative.

A brief outline answer is provided at the end of this chapter.

We should know the underpinning reasons behind that choice before we continue – particularly for groups whose choices are historically removed from their control.

Blumenthal-Barby et al. (2019) correctly note that, although the decision aids and tools of SDM encourage neutrality, the clinician can undermine that neutrality (consciously or subconsciously) with their tone, body language or language they use. They spoke about the involvement of stakeholders outside the clinician–patient relationship – infectious disease is an example of this area of practice.

Expert patients

In complex care nursing, our patients are often either experts by experience already, or are developing that expertise. In many circumstances, you are likely to be consulting with a patient or family whose expertise on one of their conditions is expert level and need to balance your knowledge with theirs. In some fields, the experts may be the family; this is particularly the case when the person themselves may not be able to advocate for themselves in all situations (due to communication or cognitive issues, or developmental abilities) (see Chapters 7, 9 and 10). For some people, such as Rosemary, the choices they must make because of their level of expertise can lead them into conflict with the services they receive.

Case study: Harry

Harry had a fall as a toddler and banged his head. For a haemophiliac this can be a major life-threatening event. Rosemary took him to the local emergency room where she was asked by a doctor how long he had had haemophilia. She made the decision to leave and drive to their specialist centre to seek treatment.

Activity 6.6   Critical thinking

What pressures would there be on Rosemary to remain at that hospital and continue with the treating team there? Assess the factors that may influence her choice.

A brief outline answer is provided at the end of this chapter.

The mechanisms and contexts of decision-making

When we pause to look at how SDM works, and who it works for, and when, we find a lot of psychological scenarios and certain contexts, mechanisms and outcomes of SDM in which it works best (Waldron et al., 2020).

Contexts

For SDM to work, three contexts are important. First, a pre-existing relationship was key – it is much easier to share the decision-making with someone you know and trust. Second, consider who you talk to when you are making decisions around important issues. How difficult the decision was to make matters: harder decisions take longer to discuss in detail. The third is health system support – rather like the House of Care, it needs to allow for time and systems in place.

Mechanisms

Waldron et al. (2020) noted several mechanisms in this process that were key. These were:

- *trust*: how much trust and confidence the person has in the other person – this goes both ways between the clinician and the patient;
- *anxiety*: the level of worry before or during the consultation. It might be about making that decision or something outside that;
- *perception of time*: the pressures of time, belief that SDM will take valuable time and the urgency of the treatment;
- *perception of other party capacity*: the belief that the other person can act in their role in the consultation. This may come from the patient since they may have doubts about the clinicians' knowledge of their condition or the treatment;
- *perception of capacity to access external support*: does the clinician believe the patient can access other sources of information?
- *world view*: beliefs, customs, values, morals, or understandings about the medical process (including religious or cultural beliefs). Again, this can come from both sides;
- *recognition of decision*: when the clinician accepts that there is a choice to be made;
- *self-efficacy*: whether the person believes they can take part in the SDM process – this includes clinicians being able to communicate their knowledge and expertise or if the patient believes they can manage that treatment.

Activity 6.7   Critical thinking

Thinking back to the information on SDM in the different specialities, does the IP-SDM work in all groups of people? What predictions might you make of barriers and adjustments you might need to make?

As this activity is based on your own thoughts, no outline answer is provided at the end of this chapter.

Embedding SDM into care

Obviously, for people living with complex needs, this is more difficult than people with a single condition. In the latter, you might have a team where SDM is the norm, and the culture accepts it. But for our person with complex needs, they might have three or four teams, spread across different organisations – that makes it much more challenging for the person.

Chapter summary

In this chapter, you have seen a glimpse of some of the reasons people with complex needs might both need SDM to be a key feature in their care and struggle with accessing it. Admittedly, SDM is not suitable for all circumstances – sometimes the situation or the person we are caring for makes it less appropriate or less desirable from the patient's viewpoint. But, even then, the option should be there and we should support our patients in this, advocating for their right to make choices with their team.

The key message that we found from researchers such as Joseph-Williams et al. (2014a) is that *skills training trumps tools for clinicians, and attitudes trump skills* (p. 2). Our attitude to shared decision-making is what makes a true difference to our patients.

In the next chapters, we will be focusing on the different areas of nursing, exploring complex needs nursing in adults, learning disabilities, mental health and children.

Activities: brief outline answers

Activity 6.5 Critical thinking (page 94)

Harriet can take a 'watch and wait' approach, attempting to provide Georgia with the information she needs as the issues arise. She could engage with a person of Georgia's nomination to act as her health advocate, making decisions and plans according to Georgia's best interests.

Activity 6.6: Critical thinking (page 95)

Rosemary might face pressures from the urgency of her son's need, against his need for quality care by a specialist team. She may face the social pressure and potential judgement of the healthcare team, leaving a department against their medical advice. She has to weigh up the risks of leaving versus staying.

Annotated further reading

The NICE guideline for shared decision-making and mental capacity: https://www.nice.org.uk/guidance/ng108

This guideline provides you with some clear understanding of legal and ethical boundaries in this area.

The MAGIC programme: evaluation: an independent evaluation of the MAGIC (making good decisions in collaboration) improvement programme. http://www.health.org.uk/sites/default/files/TheMagicProgrammeEvaluation.pdf

This gives you insights into real-world application of some of the issues discussed in this chapter.

Useful websites

https://www.nice.org.uk/guidance/ng197

The NICE guideline for SDM.

https://www.nice.org.uk/guidance/ng197/resources/shared-decision-making-learning-package-9142488109

This website takes you to the SDM learning package to support the NICE guideline on SDM.

https://www.health.org.uk/blogs/shared-decision-making-learning-from-the-boy-who-wanted-his-leg-cut-off

More information on the documentary *The Boy Who Wanted His Leg Cut Off.*

Chapter 7

Complex care in mental health

Eleri Jones

NMC Future Nurse: Standards of Proficiency for Registered Nurses

This chapter will address the following platforms and proficiencies:

Platform 3: Assessing needs and planning care

3.6 effectively assess a person's capacity to make decisions about their own care and to give or withhold consent

3.8 understand and apply the relevant laws about mental capacity for the country in which you are practising when making decisions in relation to people who do not have capacity

3.9 recognise and assess people at risk of harm and the situations that may put them at risk, ensuring prompt action is taken to safeguard those who are vulnerable

3.10 demonstrate the skills and abilities required to recognise and assess people who show signs of self-harm and/or suicidal ideation

Platform 6: Improving safety and quality of care

6.11 acknowledge the need to accept and manage uncertainty, and demonstrate an understanding of strategies that develop resilience in self and others

Platform 7: Coordinating care

7.1 understand and apply the principles of partnership, collaboration and interagency working across all relevant sectors

7.10 understand the principles and processes involved in planning and facilitating the safe discharge and transition of people between caseloads, settings and services

> ## Chapter aims
>
> ....
>
> After reading this chapter, you will be able to:
>
> - identify some of the specific issues that impact on people living with complex needs related to mental health
> - understand the mitigating factors that mental health nursing can provide to support people
> - be able to explore the types of treatments that are useful to practitioners supporting this group of patients.

Introduction

In this chapter, we will discuss complex care in people living with mental health problems (remember the definitions from Chapter 1). We will use several case studies and examples from our experts by experience to explore and apply the new concepts and revisit some introduced in the previous chapters with a mental health lens. We will examine the ways in which modern mental health nursing addresses complex health needs, and discuss capacity, consent and case management. We will explore the use of therapies and discuss some ethical issues including prescribing, treatments and communication. We will not be exploring specific conditions in terms of symptoms and treatments.

Diagnosis is a very good place to start: the most common mental health disorders include depression, anxiety, panic disorders, phobias and obsessive-compulsive disorder. We will deliberately not be going into the etiology or treatments of specific mental health disorders in this chapter but will be focusing on the external experiences and forces that act on the people living with them. Broadly, one in six people over the age of sixteen have symptoms of a mental health disorder and, more recently, this has extended to those under sixteen as well, up from one in nine in 2017 (Health Foundation, 2021). That more recent change may be related to several causes (not least Covid-19). Mental health difficulties do not occur in a vacuum, and examination of the social and political determinants of health (see Chapter 2) is necessary to see that wider picture.

Impact on physical health

According to a Public Health England analysis, people living with long-term mental illness have an increased prevalence of obesity, asthma, diabetes, chronic obstructive pulmonary disease, chronic heart disease, stroke and heart failure (Public Health England, 2018). They die an average of fifteen to twenty years earlier, and two in three deaths are from physical illnesses that can be prevented. If you add in substance misuse, the person will have some of the worse health, well-being and social outcomes. As a result of this, primary care has been incentivised to monitor people at risk, using the Quality and Outcomes Framework which provides them with additional payments to do yearly checks of blood pressure, glucose, cholesterol and body mass index (Kendrick, 2014). It should include the use of alcohol, drugs and smoking, as well as cervical screening (where appropriate). In some practices, they may use waist circumference as a measure too since BMI is often criticised as a reliable measurement of health. This can result in a comprehensive care plan, made with the person and their support network (Kendrick, 2014).

Definitions

There is no easy test for mental health – we have questionnaires, scans and blood tests to exclude other causes but primarily use the ICD-11 (World Health Organization, 2018) with some referring to the DSM (American Psychiatric Association, 2022). It is one of those rare areas of practice where there is a clear definition of complex needs. This is provided by the All Party Parliamentary Group on Complex Needs and Dual Diagnosis and created by a broad group of stakeholders (All Party Parliamentary Group on Complex Needs and Dual Diagnosis, 2014). This group, which focuses exclusively on addiction and mental health, defines complex needs as someone with two or more needs affecting their physical, mental, social, or financial well-being.

Box 7.1 The All Party Parliamentary Group on Complex Needs and Dual Diagnosis Definition

People with complex needs must have two or more of the following:

- mental health issues
- substance misuse issues
- dual diagnosis of mental health and substance misuse issues
- physical health condition
- a learning disability
- a history of offending behaviour
- a physical disability
- employment problems
- homelessness or housing issues
- family or relationship difficulties
- domestic violence
- social isolation
- poverty
- trauma (physical, psychological, or social).

(All Party Parliamentary Group on Complex Needs and Dual Diagnosis, 2014)

They note that these needs can be severe, longstanding, difficult to diagnose and therefore difficult to treat (All Party Parliamentary Group on Complex Needs and Dual Diagnosis, 2014). Manning and Gagnon (2017) noted that there is a good transferability of this definition to the broader discussions in healthcare. But look at how many of these relate to the social and political determinants of health (Chapter 3)? It becomes harder to separate people living with complex needs from the broader picture, particularly if we are to avoid individualising the issue of complex needs in mental health (The King's Fund, 2019a).

Social and political determinants

Having explored this a little in previous chapters, it becomes obvious that stable employment and housing contribute massively to mental illness, but there are other determinants (see Chapter 3 for an in-depth discussion) (NHS England, 2016).

- Groups like veterans with mental health problems, marginalised groups and older people are less diagnosed and less likely to be treated.
- As many as nine out of ten people in prison have a mental health, drug, or alcohol problem.
- Survivors of domestic violence often find their care medicalised.
- Black people were four times more likely to be detained under the Mental Health Act and diagnosed with a mental illness in systems such as the criminal justice system (40 per cent), rather than the health system. They are more likely to be diagnosed with schizophrenia (six to eighteen-fold elevated rate), compared to the general population (1 per cent of the population).

(NHS England, 2016; Walker, 2020)

In Chapter 2, we highlighted the difficult choices people must make around their finances and we discussed social and political determinants of health in Chapter 3. There is a 65 per cent employment gap for those being seen by secondary mental health services compared to the general population and they are often in low-pay, high-turnover jobs that are part time or temporary.

Activity 7.1 Reflection

Take a moment and imagine that you knew you would have enough money to be housed, fed, warm and cover your bills forever. What do you feel? Compare that to the discussions around the choices people must make and consider how you might feel in that situation instead?

As this activity is based on your own reflection, no outline answer is provided at the end of the chapter.

You can see from this exercise the reasons that would need holistic assessment and the potential impact on mental health. We need to consider our practice, ensuring that it includes their experiences, challenges and any trauma that they have faced before in the broader picture.

Trauma-informed care

Adverse childhood events (ACEs) are things that happen before the age of eighteen which may be potentially traumatic such as abuse or neglect, domestic violence and so on. This trauma may impact people for the rest of their lives; we need to be mindful in mental health that many people living with mental health problems have experienced traumatic events, whether it be before or after the age of eighteen. Some of them may have been at the hands of those who could have been reasonably expected to act in a professional, caring manner (i.e., healthcare professionals). When we provide trauma-informed care, we create an environment where a person who has been through trauma can feel safe and trust those around them. Sensitivity to questioning, mindfulness over locations of care, and so on avoids excluding someone who has received trauma from those services (The King's Fund, 2019b).

Sweeney et al. (2016) cite the large evidence base for the link between trauma and mental health. The role of political and social determinants of health has been discussed before in this book (Chapter 3) and most certainly applies here but Sweeney et al. go on to discuss retraumatisation, a process where someone experiences something that triggers the same emotional and physiological responses. Remember the story of Bettie in the previous chapters, where she felt her life would have been greatly improved had someone addressed her trauma? This can happen in mental health services; women's responses to domestic violence being treated as hysteria, responses to racism as an individual problem, or homosexuality or queerness as something in need of corrective treatment (Sweeney et al., 2016).

Box 7.2   Key principles of trauma-informed approaches

1. Recognise the prevalence, signs and impacts of trauma
2. Resist retraumatisation
3. Consider cultural, historical and gender contexts
4. Trustworthiness and transparency
5. Collaboration and mutuality
6. Empowerment, choice and control
7. Safety
8. Survivor partnerships
9. Pathways to trauma-specific care.

(Sweeney et al., 2016, p. 178)

Similarly, Guest (2021) identified four attributes – recognition, knowledge, concern and respect – which defined trauma-informed care (Figure 7.1). In these, the clinician must recognise that the trauma exists, which in Bettie's case had not happened. Think back to Chapter 4, where we discussed this issue. If the first step is the ability to recognise the trauma, then it is vital that our communication with our patients be open to the idea that more is happening for them in that moment than is happening for us. They may not be able to identify the source of their emotions, or acknowledge their own trauma, which adds complexity to the situation. They may choose not to disclose or feel unsafe to do so. As clinicians, we have an ethical duty of care to our patients, and part of that includes an awareness of what has happened to them and how that is working within their lives now.

Case study: Bettie's perspective

(In Bettie's own words – contains some distressing content around sexual abuse.)

In my experience this is the case.

I first disclosed to my GP that I had been sexually abused as a child in 1999, some twenty years after the event. I was experiencing symptoms of depression with poor sleep, tearfulness and flashbacks. I was referred to a psychiatrist and a psychologist and, despite numerous references to my childhood sexual abuse and the use of the word 'trauma' in my medical notes, nobody seemed to be joining the dots. Instead, I was given various diagnostic labels over the following tortuous years of borderline personality disorder, cyclothymia, bipolar disorder, severe depression and moderate depression. The personality disorder diagnosis was written into my notes without it being discussed with me and despite the fact that I quite clearly did not meet the criteria for having it!

I was medicated with numerous anti-psychotics and anti-depressants which in my opinion exacerbated my symptoms. The damaging label of personality disorder was left attached to me as a diagnosis for over ten years until I successfully challenged it with the help of an independent psychiatrist who agreed that I never met the criteria for that diagnosis and that it had been damaging to my healthcare.

Activity 7.2   Reflection

Read Bettie's story and consider how that might impact someone like her. What would change if a healthcare professional was able to help her work through her emotional trauma from the abuse early in her story? How did her story impact on her relationship with healthcare professionals?

As this activity is based on your own reflection, no outline answer is provided at the end of the chapter.

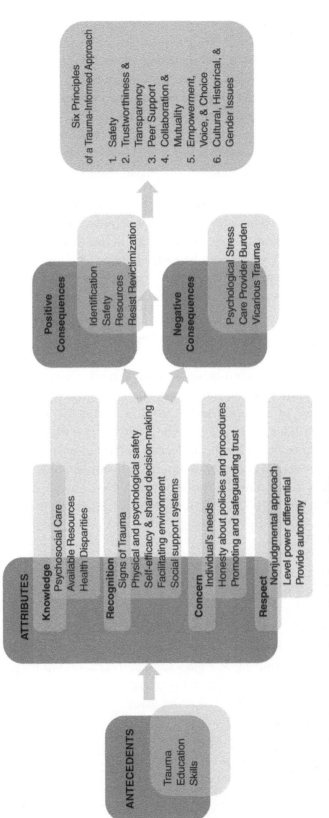

Figure 7.1 Trauma-informed care (based on Guest, 2021)

Communication

Communication is vital in all parts of nursing but those living with mental health issues rated effective communication, with empathy and compassion, as a sought-after trait in their nurses (Horgan et al., 2021). The importance of these highlights the need for your own therapeutic skills in communication to be strong. Abdolrahimi et al. (2017, p. 4973) stated that these *therapeutic skills are an important means in building interpersonal relationships, a process of information transmission, an important clinical competency, a structure with two different sections* and *a significant tool in patient centred care.*

Body language is well known to be a large part of communication; try and think of an appointment you have been to where the person's focus was on the form in front of them. Being aware of your body language is useful in day-to-day communication but it increases in importance if you are working with someone who is hearing voices or experiencing paranoia (Bowers et al., 2009).

Pharmacotherapy and ethics

Treatments in mental health often bring up ethical questions, such as indications for treatment, risks, benefits and alternative management strategies (Beck et al., 2021). Our ethical position is often supported or guided by the rule of law, including case law and legal frameworks such as the Mental Capacity Act – what is legal for us to do, in terms of restricting someone's right to leave a building or enforcing a line of treatment. Often, we must make choices between the available options, some of which have a serious, undesirable result. Equally, the least restrictive principle can result in positive outcomes, where the person is safe but not overly restricted. We therefore have several guiding principles to work with.

Box 7.3 Ethical principles

- Respect for persons: regard for an individual's worth and dignity
- Autonomy: self-governance
- Beneficence: the responsibility to act in a way that seeks to provide the greatest benefit
- Fidelity: faithfulness to the interests of the patient
- Non-maleficence: the commitment to do no harm
- Veracity: the duty of truth and honesty
- Justice: the act of fair treatment, without prejudice
- Privacy: protection of patients' personal information
- Integrity: honourable conduct within the profession.

(Beck et al., 2021)

You might think these are clear and obvious, but the history of healthcare shows us that they are often breached. Debates on ethical choices happen all the time, and you often see legal cases where two sides cannot agree on what is both ethical and legal, such Wye Valley NHS Trust v B [2015], which focused on the person's ability to agree to the amputation of his leg, or Kings College Hospital NHS Foundation Trust v C [2015], where the person did not wish to receive treatment to save their life after attempting suicide (General Medical Council, 2020). Therefore, our own actions should be well reasoned and evidence-based, often made alongside our patient and with the MDT.

Capacity and the Mental Capacity Act (2005)

The ability to make decisions for yourself is known as 'capacity'; we have a basic right to make our own choices, without influence or pressure (Peisah, 2017). We have a duty to consider capacity only if there is doubt – that is, you should have a reason to question their capacity. It is decision-specific; I may have capacity to decide what to eat and what to wear but not to give my house away.

The principles of the Mental Capacity Act 2005

The following principles apply for the purposes of this Act.

1. A person must be assumed to have capacity unless it is established that he lacks capacity.
2. A person is not to be treated as unable to make a decision unless all practicable steps to help him to do so have been taken without success.
3. A person is not to be treated as unable to make a decision merely because he makes an unwise decision.
4. An act done, or decision made, under this Act for or on behalf of a person who lacks capacity must be done, or made, in his best interests.
5. Before the act is done, or the decision is made, regard must be had to whether the purpose for which it is needed can be as effectively achieved in a way that is less restrictive of the person's rights and freedom of action.

(Hubbard and Stone, 2018, p. 8)

The reasons someone may not have capacity to make a decision are wide ranging, from temporary conditions to long-term issues, age or learning disabilities (see Chapters 9 and 10 for information around learning disabilities and children). The point of establishing capacity is often to consider if someone can make a choice around their treatment (or rejection of treatment), as well as other legal decisions.

Critiques of the Mental Capacity Act 2005

The United Nations Convention on the Rights of Persons with Disabilities does reject the functional tests, suggesting instead that 'will and preferences' replace it, at least as a first point (Donnelly, 2016). These functional tests require that the person has:

- the ability to retain the information long enough to make the decision;
- the ability to use, or 'weigh up' the information as part of the decision-making process; and
- the ability to communicate their decision through any means.

(Hardy and Joyce, 2009)

They argue that there are no circumstances in which the person's will and preferences should be denied. Donnelly (2016) links these concepts to dignity, as to deny them is to ignore the personhood of a person, and argue that to deny autonomy is to undermine a person's dignity. Coggon (2016) suggests that the issue is not binary – that a person does or does not have capacity. They suggest that there is a difference between those who lack capacity but have made their wishes and values known, and those who have not done so. This suggestion gives a greater value to the patient's preferences and will, especially when they are written down in advance of the current episode of care.

Consent

For consent to be truly given, it must be given without persuasion or coercion (Department of Health, 2009). It should be given as informed consent with the information that person needs provided to them.

There are specific areas where you might need to consider capacity as part of consent, in that a person without capacity may not be able to consent to treatment or to be part of a research study. The person has the right to autonomy, respect for will and preferences, and supported decision-making provision. They have a right to access healthcare, even if they are unable to consent; refusing if they do not have capacity is not a reason to deny them the right to treatment but the decisions should be made in their best interests (Department of Health, 2009).

Box 7.4   Case law

There are two cases in law that illustrate this delicate balance.

Re C (adult: refusal of treatment) [1994] 1 All ER 819
C, the patient, was detained in hospital and had paranoid schizophrenia but had developed gangrene. He declined the proposed removal of his leg repeatedly and it went to

court, with the hospital stating that his capacity to make that choice was impaired by his illness and that he did not understand the risk of death. The court found that, although his general capacity was impaired, he understood and was able to retain the specific information and had arrived at a choice. He therefore had capacity to make that specific decision (and it turned out alright in the end!).

Re T (adult: refusal of medical treatment) [2004] 3 All ER 387

T, a young woman with a history of self-harming which had led to dangerously low haemoglobin levels, refused a blood transfusion. She believed her blood was evil and that receiving the transfusion would increase the *danger of my committing acts of evil*. The court decision was that she was unable to use or weigh up the information or the factors in making that decision and therefore she did not have capacity.

Activity 7.3   Reflection

Consider your own future; are there treatments you would decline or prefer? Find a local framework for advance care planning in mental health and try to complete it for yourself. You might consider treatments such as medication, hospitalisation or electro-convulsive therapy and document your preferences around them.

What might change those preferences?

As this activity is based on your own reflection, no outline answer is provided at the end of the chapter.

This seems clear cut, doesn't it? We all know that consent is required for any treatment. One important fact is that to give consent, you must have capacity to do so (but see more about Gillick competency and Fraser guidelines in young people in Chapter 10).

Unfortunately, in a survey with healthcare professionals, Lamont et al. (2019) demonstrated that some of them did not understand consent and decision-making capacity. Although this is a small sample (n = 86), it does show that thorough and well-documented decision processes are vital, as is a good knowledge of the legal frameworks around consent and capacity. Availability and access to appropriate care is a large part of receiving the correct treatment, at the right time and in the best place.

Funding Mental Health in the NHS

In 2012, the Health and Social Care Act required that the NHS deliver 'parity of esteem' between mental and physical health services, an achievement that was intended to be completed by 2020. What this means is that the focus of the NHS should be on improving both physical and mental health equally. This built on the mental health strategy published in 2011. But for context, although mental health accounts for 23 per cent of the burden of disease, it receives 11 per cent of the NHS budget. It experienced the second largest cut in acute beds at 73 per cent between 1987 and 2020, with the intent to provide more care in the community (The King's Fund, 2015). This has resulted in an increase in people being moved to different areas if they need a bed, making it harder for their relatives and friends to provide support (Royal College of Psychiatrists, 2019). It received multiple cuts that impacted the ability of staff to deliver care in the community, moving from a case management model to one where people received treatments and were then discharged back to their GP's care (The King's Fund, 2021).

It is worth noting that mental health funding has not been ring-fenced by the government or NHS England; this means that (in England at least) the local commissioners can decide how much to spend on mental health services, sometimes resulting in a postcode lottery. The NHS Long-Term Plan does include some ring-fenced funds by 2023 (Baker, 2021) and NHS England (2016) sets out a delivery plan for the Five Year Plan by 2020–1 including increasing the funding for mental health and ring-fencing it. It is highly probable that the impact of the pandemic has caused issues with this.

Access

Another issue for people with complex needs living in the community is access to talking therapy; there are long waiting times (Baker, 2021). Remember that each area sets out their own funding levels for mental health: this results in a 'postcode lottery' for access to therapies and specialist services. Waiting times for talking therapies are on average 21 days until the first treatment and then 53 days until their second treatment (see Figure 7.2).

When you examine this more locally during 2020–1, in Essex, the waiting time was four days, whereas in Bristol, North Somerset and South Gloucestershire, it was 86 days (see Figure 7.2). Although these services are often targeted at early intervention of depression and anxiety, this delay impacts on those living with complex needs. Remember from the previous chapters that those living with physical complex needs may develop anxiety and depression.

Case study: Charlotte

Charlotte is a cisgender woman, aged 34. She lives with her partner in a flat owned by a housing association. She is employed in a local supermarket for a few hours a week but does not have a fixed contract. Her partner is employed as a driver and is often away overnight. She does not have family support around her and has a few friends in the local area.

In the last six months, she has found that she has become very depressed and is struggling to get out of bed. She has found herself avoiding leaving the home and has started to forget things.

IAPT average waiting times, 2020/21

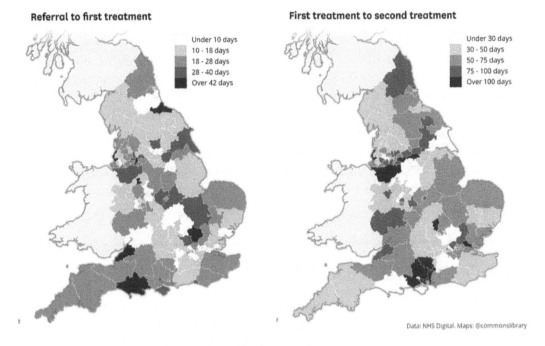

Figure 7.2   IAPT average waiting times (Baker, 2021).

Activity 7.4   Critical thinking

Thinking critically, consider the social and political determinants of health that might be contributing to Charlotte's situation. What impact might the waiting times for the local talking therapies have on her?

A brief outline answer is given at the end of the chapter.

Even after being seen by a service, people often felt that they needed more time or more support before being discharged back to the care of their GP – in an examination of experiences of 13,000 adult service users, only 43 per cent in 2018 felt they had seen NHS Mental Health Services enough for their needs (National Institute for Health and Care Excellence, 2019). In areas where waiting lists are high, people will wait for a longer period; the shorter waiting time to treatment results in better outcomes for the person (NHS England, 2021). There are a number of different models of care within the health service, and we will explore three of them.

Models of care

Broadly, most of the focus of mental health integrated care MDT work is often around older people living with complexities such as dementia. You will find specialist nurses being placed in GP practices as part of a front line, early intervention model. There are crisis teams, which focus on short-term stabilisation, and recovery teams, which are longer term. Expansion of improving access to psychological therapies (IAPT) programmes is a key part of the recent changes to the health service. You may also see social prescribing in GP or primary care services. When mental health services were examined by the King's Fund, by talking to over 100 people involved in a broad range of mental health services in both urban and city locations, from staff to experts by experience, it found differences in perspective, hostility and distrust at times (The King's Fund, 2019a).

Stepped care models

Many of those living with complex mental health needs are likely to meet the crisis and the recovery teams in particular. Anthony defines the concept of 'recovery' in mental health as *living a satisfying, hopeful and contributing life even with the limitations caused by illness* (cited by Naylor et al., 2017, p. 29). The aim is to bring the expertise of mental health staff into the teams that encounter people living with complexity, rather than having it as a separate service; this might look like having mental health specialists placed in primary care (Naylor et al., 2017). As you can see in Figure 7.3, the levels of care reflect a similar style to that in physical health, moving from whole population to highly complex needs, with consideration for the issues that might be impacting on that person such as social determinants of health (Furst et al., 2018). Stepped care aims to provide the right level of treatment at the right time, moving a person through the levels of service up to intensive, according to their need. This is the model used by IAPT models, with clinical assessments used to decide which level to place a person on. Earlier in the chapter, we discussed the waiting times for services like this and it is worthy of note that according to NHS England (2016) only 14 per cent of people felt they received the right response in crisis.

Case management

Much of the information from Chapter 5 around case management applies to mental health as well as other areas of practice. In mental health, we see a combination of approaches to work with service users, including care coordination, trying to reduce the impact of the person's ill health on their lives, reducing admissions and so forth. But in mental health, we might see types of case management where the person with complex needs may not be as willing or able to engage. This is known as assertive community treatment or outreach and tends to focus on the people who we think need the

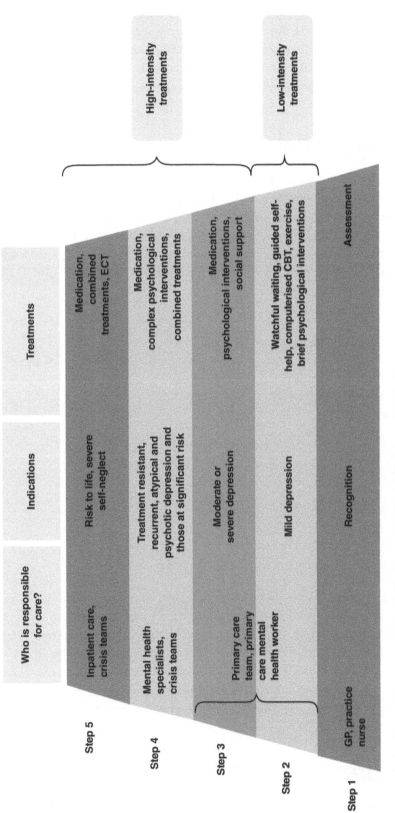

Figure 7.3 Stepped care models (KCE Reports 265, 2016, ©kce.fgov.be)

most help. The visits tend to be in the person's home or other locations outside the health system. It is an MDT approach and is not a service where people are limited by the amount of time that they remain supported by the team or by traditional working-week boundaries. An evolution of this is known as intensive case management. Both have been found to reduce hospital admissions (Dieterich et al., 2017).

Recovery model

The recovery model focuses on stability and building resilience; this is often linked to wellness recovery action plans (WRAP) created with the person involved around hope, personal responsibility, education, self-advocacy and support (The King's Fund, 2019a). Similarly, the Recovery Star measures resilience in ten areas of life; the fourth edition was created using feedback from mental health professionals, organisations, commissioners and service users and acknowledged that self-reliance is not always a possible or appropriate goal for some people.

Box 7.5   Recovery Star

- Managing mental health
- Physical health and self-care
- Trust and hope
- Living skills
- Social networks
- Work
- Relationships
- Addictive behaviour
- Responsibilities
- Identity and self esteem

But the King's Fund (2019a) found that some staff expressed frustration that contracts pushed certain goals onto the team and the service users, such as smoking cessation and weight loss. They cite service users, clinicians, voluntary organisations and academics who suggest that the narrowness of health outcomes and definitions of wellness remove the model from the holistic design towards a more mechanical approach. This is strongly linked to the commissioning approach: think back to the House of Care (Figure 5.3) and the importance of designing services around the needs of service users.

Crisis care

Dalton-Locke et al. (2021) identified a range of crisis services across the UK, many of which have not provided evidence of their models. Of particular concern are models such as the Serenity Integrated Mentoring model, which worked with police to reduce emergency service use. This has faced criticisms about the ethical issues with police involvement during crisis and the potential harm from encouraging someone not to seek help in this way. Models such as the crisis café, safe havens or recovery cafés are growing despite the lack of efficacy, whereas acute day units, which have strong evidence supporting them, seem to be reducing. The former is often provided by the voluntary sector, while the latter is usually NHS. The importance of evidence-based practice should not be ignored in service design, however well meaning.

Integrated care

The King's Fund (2017) explored the integrated approaches to mental health in the vanguard sites (West Cheshire Way MCP and Tower Hamlets Together MCP), finding that the cross-work between staff members allowed them to ask for help informally and increased the work with the voluntary sector. You can see this in the work by Ratzliff et al. (2016) where the strategies within the team revolved around the ability to share care and communicate. This might include goal-sharing, trust, clear roles and workflow, and communication strategies. They explored accountable practice, which includes the need for goals, measurements to be decided and progress reviewed. Within all their work they are putting the patient in the centre as part of this team. Scenarios such as Gemma's are common, with the patient's goals placed first in the care planning process, which requires delicate communication.

Case study: Gemma

Gemma, who takes long-term antipsychotic medication for her bipolar disorder, is struggling with her weight gain. Exercise is a challenge because it requires her to go to a new place and she feels self-conscious of her size and her lack of knowledge of the machines.

Activity 7.5   Critical thinking

Assuming you were her care coordinator, explore your local area for activities you might be able to signpost her to that might be less daunting for her. What might you need to consider for her personal preferences, financial or social situation?

A brief outline answer is given at the end of the chapter.

With all treatments, a person should provide informed consent to receive it, whether it be medication, talking therapies or other interventions. They must be balanced with the best available evidence and the clinician's expert knowledge.

The triangle of care

This is a specific standard to address some key problems found in children and young people mental health services (CYPMHS) but is used in adult services now. It stems from the need to acknowledge support for carers and families, to build resilience in children and young people and support self-care (Carers Trust, 2020). It introduced six standards (see below).

Box 7.6   Triangle of care

- Standard 1: Carers and their essential role are identified at first contact or as soon as possible afterwards
- Standard 2: Staff are carer aware and trained in carer engagement strategies
- Standard 3: Policy and practice protocols re: confidentiality and sharing information, [sic] are in place
- Standard 4: Defined post(s) responsible for carers are in place
- Standard 5: A carer introduction to the service and staff is available, with a relevant range of information across the care pathway
- Standard 6: A range of carer support is available.

(Carers Trust, 2020)

Diagnosis of exclusion

Although we have specifically focused on experiences and context of living with mental health problems, we have avoided talking about individual diagnosis at depth. But we cannot avoid addressing the issue of diagnoses that might cause people to be excluded from services for being too complex or other such terms. That is borderline personality disorder (BPD) or emotionally unstable personality disorder (EUPD) but may include complex emotional needs (Sheridan Rains et al., 2021). Perkins et al. (2018) found that this diagnosis carried the most institutionalised stigma and was most likely to cause removal of services, despite repeated insistence that it is not a diagnosis of exclusion. Warrender et al. (2021) found accessing help in a crisis was difficult, tending to be reactive instead of proactive in managing risk. They cite studies showing that lack of collaboration impacted their care, with 65.4 per cent experiencing discrimination from healthcare professionals. In better news, Sheridan Rains et al. (2021) found that there was an increase in services for this diagnosis; unfortunately, they still struggled to get good-quality treatment in the community. To receive professionalism, clinical knowledge, respect, compassion, effective interventions and positive/non-stigmatising attitudes from professionals is not an unreasonable ask and should be a baseline of care (Sheridan Rains et al., 2021). The most positive qualities in healthcare professionals often came from those specially trained in this area.

People living with mental illness often find that interactions with healthcare professionals can result in feeling excluded from decisions, receiving threats of coercive treatment, long waiting times, lack of information or being treated in a paternalistic manner (Knaak et al., 2017). Professionals have used language such as difficult, manipulative, or non-compliant to describe people living with mental illness (The King's Fund, 2019a). Although we wish healthcare professionals were excluded from stigmatising our patients, there is a long history of evidence suggesting the opposite (Ahmedani, 2011). Stigma is when we take an attribute and reduce someone to a tainted, discounted person because of it, whether it be race, gender, sexual orientation, or illness (Ahmedani, 2011); evidence suggests that we carry the same stigmas as the general population, and that our patients can feel as excluded, stigmatised and labelled as anyone. This is particularly relevant for people living with complex needs in mental health since they are often experiencing situations where stigma may be applied by broader society.

It is vital that we be aware of our own biases and values and begin to work through those. The barriers created by stigma can deny a person much-needed support and can be at two different levels: person-level and provider- and system-level (Corrigan et al., 2014). Personal change is necessary and understanding stigma is an excellent place to start with that; we receive training, and it is clear how we should act. But where stigma is perpetuated, change is essential. Think about the availability of services we spoke about earlier in the chapter – without services, help-seeking is impossible (Corrigan et al., 2014).

Conclusion

Throughout this chapter, we have tried to make the point that the patient must have autonomy, choice and respect in their care. Awareness of the stigma and previous experiences the person may have had with healthcare is vital in working with this group of patients, as is awareness of the legal and ethical issues.

Chapter summary

In this chapter, we have discussed legalities, ethics and treatments for people living with complex care needs. Specifically, we have looked at capacity and consent. We have explored the systems and power, and how their previous experiences may impact their current situation. We have looked at a range of models of care, including recovery, integrated care, care coordination, stepped care and crisis care. We hope that we have, throughout the chapter, emphasised the need to treat the person with respect and consider their preferences and autonomy.

Activities: brief outline answers

Activity 7.4 Critical thinking (page 111)

Charlotte lives in a housing association property (environment, community safety) and has uncertain employment (economic status, food, inequality) and therefore income. She is isolated without support (community safety, demographics).

With a delay in talking therapies, the time when she is willing and able to engage may pass. There may be an increased risk of her mental health deteriorating further, relationships breaking down or impact on her employment.

Activity 7.5 Critical thinking (page 115)

You might find community groups, mental health support groups, activities that she would enjoy, or physical exercise like group walking.

You would need to consider her interests and dislikes. You would also need to consider the cost of travel and the activity, or the level of personal contact she can manage at that time. You would need to consider the useable hours she has and the impact on her employment.

Annotated further reading

Egan, G. (2013) *The Skilled Helper: A Problem-Management and Opportunity-Development Approach to Helping.* Andover: Cengage Learning.

Highlights the use of self as a therapeutic tool.

Lamont, S., Stewart, C. and Chiarella, M. (2019) Capacity and consent: knowledge and practice of legal and healthcare standards. *Nursing Ethics*, 26(1), 71–83.

This article will support your understanding of the key issues around capacity and consent.

Useful websites

http://www.acestudy.org

The ACE Study gives you some insight to the impact of childhood experiences on a person's health and well-being as an adult.

MIND: http://www.mind.org.uk

Rethink: http://www.rethink.org

National Elf Service: https://www.nationalelfservice.net/

These sites are good, reliable, accessible information with signposting.

Chapter 8   Complex care in adults

Introduction

Throughout this book, we have discussed issues and examples of complex care needs and the nursing considerations. In this chapter, we are going to focus on adult nursing and explore complex care nursing in adults. Specifically, we are going to connect the broader concepts in relation to some familiar and some new case studies. We will discuss some new concepts around energy management and sensitive topics of discussion.

Statistics

There are some clear numbers on the percentage of LTCs in those aged 60+; there are 58 per cent living with a single LTC in the UK, which drops to 25 per cent with two or more, with the percentages mirroring the age as they rise (Frost et al., 2020). This often excludes conditions such as frailty, dementia, Parkinson's disease, or stroke, which are common in older people, or mental health conditions such as depression. Despite this, the level of adults living with complex care needs is unknown, partially because there is an overlap with people with LTCs, but also because, by their very definition, the systems we have do not work to meet their needs and we have a fragmented view of their lives and needs.

Guidelines

The NICE guidelines for *Older People with Social Care Needs and Multiple Long-term Conditions* (2015) focuses on actions when someone has more than one LTC, once again putting the illness above the person in the process, despite the drive for person-centric care. As you have seen throughout the book, for people living with complex needs, it is vital that they are centred and are the person driving the direction of the care they receive. Using strategies and setting goals do little unless they are suitable for that individual. Throughout the book, we hope we have made it clear that they face issues where their needs meet the functions and systems of health and social care.

Energy theories

One issue we have not discussed is that of energy and the impact that has on the person's ability to engage in decision-making processes, self-management and self-care, as well as on the rest of their lives. For this, allow me to introduce you to the Unified Cutlery Theory; this is a theory that combines three others (Spoon Theory (Miserandino, 2003), Fork Theory (Rose, 2018) and Knife Theory (Masson, 2019)). The aim of these theories was to express the issues around energy use for people with chronic conditions and that is something vital for you to grasp if you are to care for your patients with complex needs. This is particularly the case for invisible conditions where the impact can be felt but not often seen.

Spoon Theory

The spoon is a unit of energy. If you have eight spoons for the day, and you have a number of tasks to complete, each task will take X number of spoons. These spoons can be emotional, mental or physical, or any combination of all of them. Spoon numbers will vary for people – one day, you may wake with a dozen and the next only three, sometimes for no clear reason. Imagine having eight spoons and knowing that your personal hygiene will take up four of those, but you must make several phone calls (heavy on the emotional spoons!) and wash the dishes. This hopefully demonstrates that, sometimes, our patients must make hard choices about what they do with their spoons, which are recovered by quality rest, which can be difficult to come by if you have high pain or anxiety levels. You can save up spoons but that requires restricting activity before and after.

Fork Theory

Forks are stresses; imagine having forks stuck into you and consider how that may make things worse. A fork might be financial stress, relationship issues or anything that makes you feel worse or things to be a little harder. When the limit of forks that can be tolerated is hit, a person may not be able to handle anything more. Forks can be varying in size – from small forks to pitchforks, and they can prevent use of spoons.

Knife Theory

Knives come into play when you have run out of spoons or have too many forks stuck in you to reach for them, but you have, for one reason or other, to keep going. A knife is an overdraft – energy taken from the future, taking a person beyond safe limits.

Jagged Spoons

A newer addition to the cutlery drawer is the jagged spoon; this is a tool that allows you to function as if you had a spoon but hurts you as if it were a knife. It may be a medication, a mood or a symptom of your condition that allows you to step on, putting off the pain that you will experience to the next day.

Unified Cutlery Theory

By bringing these together, we have the Unified Cutlery Theory, providing us with language to understand the experience of people living with complex needs with energy limitations. This language, developed initially to allow an able-bodied person to understand the importance placed by those with chronic or complex conditions on their time, allows us to grasp the importance of what we are asking. When we ask our patients to engage in the processes we think would be valuable, we are asking them to use spoons, as a minimum. Self-managing medications, when they might be taking thirteen different ones a day, is a large task, as is organising appointments or balancing two conditions where the specialists are not working together. Equally, advocating for themselves is exhausting and fighting the current way the health and social care system works is a perpetual drip-feed of spoons. A phone call to book an appointment, for example, might be equal to the number of spoons required to perform a vital self-care task. The original author of the Spoon Theory explains her reason for developing it here:

> *The difference in being sick and being healthy is having to make choices or to consciously think about things when the rest of the world doesn't have to. The healthy have the luxury of a life without choices, a gift most people take for granted [...] I used spoons to convey this point. [...] If I was in control of taking away the spoons, then she would know what it feels like to have someone or something else, in this case, Lupus, being in control.*

> (Miserandino, 2003, n.p.)

The idea is not only about energy then but also around loss – loss of control, loss of function and loss of a life without choices between things that matter.

Activity 8.1   Reflection

Considering the quote above, reflect on a situation in your life where you had to make this type of difficult choice or (if you have been lucky enough not to have that situation) reflect on a recent patient you have cared for. Consider the grief they may have experienced in having to make that choice.

As this activity is based on your own reflection, no outline answer is provided at the end of this chapter.

Grief and loss are often themes in adults living with complex needs – even if those needs have been with them since childhood (as with Harry), it is normal for them to experience periods of strong emotions when comparing to peers or when letting go of something they loved doing because of the new limitations. This can impact on engagement with services; Michlig et al. (2018) found that the services that considered those issues and included mental health support had higher levels of engagement.

Bringing those issues together, you may be able to see why care coordination (Chapters 4, 5, 7, 9 and 10) becomes a key foundation for support for adults with complex care needs. In the scenario below, Colette demonstrates how she must navigate tasks which we might take for granted, and how fighting the system adds to the energy drain. Furthermore, engaging with a system that represents something you have strong feelings around takes more energy – to make or attend appointments that represent loss, anger or grief is harder than it might otherwise be.

Case study: Colette

This is in her own words:

Although I have a good GP whenever I was referred to a consultant, they almost always said I had tendonitis and put it down to rheumatoid arthritis. This never quite fitted as my x-rays were too good – i.e., no bone deterioration considering the length of time I had trouble. Physios gave up as I got worse rather than better with their treatment. When in my early 50s a few things came together and I was diagnosed by a rheumatologist as having EDS, thank goodness! She picked up on it very quickly, in fact as I was walking into the consulting room; obviously further investigations confirmed the diagnosis and I have never looked back since and everything fitted into place and as time has gone on quite a few other things from my childhood fitted into the picture.

As life goes on, I manage reasonably well despite getting worse as my body ages. If I relied on social services I would be housebound, having ready-prepared food delivered to the door – to save me struggling in the supermarket and the practicalities of cooking from my wheelchair; my NHS wheelchair does not go well outside and I cannot cook when sitting in my chair as the kitchen units are higher than I am which is a health and safety issue – there is a simple solution, put an extra motor on the chair that will rise me up, but cooking and eating is a social need not a mobility problem. I do hope that going forwards different services are integrated thus finding all-round solutions that fit the person and not just the cheapest common solution. There have been some professionals that have been very good and considerate of my problems, but it often is the 'system' that is at fault.

Over the years I have spent a fortune on equipment that works for me; it has been hard particularly as household income was minimal, but the sacrifice of other activities and holidays made a better life for all of us. I wear braces on most of my joints which give support while at the same time allow for full but not over movement (as opposed to splints which stop a joint from moving); again NHS issue are not good enough, so I have purchased my own that work better.

When you explore cases such as Colette's you can see she had trouble getting to a diagnosis, and that struggle alone takes up energy and time. She speaks about the difficulties she has accessing the solutions she needs through our health and social care systems, and the challenges of purchasing her own equipment.

Activity 8.2   Critical thinking

Reading the scenario above, where might the system be adjusted to provide Colette with tools that would reduce energy drain?

A brief outline answer is provided at the end of this chapter.

You can see how the social and financial determinants of health (Figure 2.1) play into Colette's life – purchasing equipment instead of holidays or other activities becomes a priority. Have a look at some of the potential impacts of parenting children (Chapter 10) and apply those thoughts to the situation for adults. Wheelchairs are an ideal example; the ones provided by the NHS may not suit the needs of many adults (lightweight) or adapt to the situations they would like to experience (off-road or festivals or fairs, for example). When we return to the House of Care model (Figure 5.3) and recall the criticisms of that model, Colette's situation is well situated to demonstrate the problems with that division; separating health and social care means that needs which straddle the two fall into the gap. Therefore, when we consider the models of working such as our example complex care teams, which can work to bridge that gap, you can see some of the benefits to our patients instantly. Without that, Colette is responsible for working between the two, finding a solution and advocating for herself or purchasing her own equipment.

Activity 8.3   Team working

When considering Colette's scenario, imagine you are in the complex care team; which team members would you think essential to her assessment, and what priorities do you hear from her story? How would those team members work together to achieve the goals Colette is setting?

A brief outline answer is provided at the end of this chapter.

It is important to consider the impact of this energy drain on other aspects of life. Think back to the Roper–Logan–Tierney model of nursing (Figure 4.1), and remember that working, playing and expressing sexuality are parts of that – often neglected parts, admittedly, but as humans we need that social interaction and contact.

Case study: Colette

This is in her own words:

I do have a 24-hour carer – he is an invaluable canine partner, a dog that assists me with many physical tasks: opening and closing the fridge and other doors; carrying things like my large bath sheet into the bathroom; passes things to me; gets the washing out of the washing machine; picks up dropped items; gets food off supermarket shelves; pulls undone the Velcro on my braces and gets me completely undressed just to mention a few things. All this work that he does saves stress on my joints and now I am living alone there is companionship; and just as importantly I have to look after him by feeding, grooming, exercising, playing etc. but it is a small price to pay for his help and it helps to keep me going.

As you can see, Colette has found ways to support herself with a living companion, and the balance of energies here is important to note – although he requires output of her energy, he equally saves her energy. Importantly, he is her partner, working with her in her life (a very well trained one!).

Activity 8.4   Critical thinking

Considering the role of Colette's companion, can you think of other circumstances in health where animals have been used to support people with complex needs? Consider how people can access that 'service' – these animals are highly trained experts and that requires a considerable investment.

A brief outline answer is provided at the end of this chapter.

One thing that is often isolated throughout the case studies our experts have kindly shared with us is the isolation that complex needs can cause. This is not purely related to the needs themselves, or the mismatch with the health and social care system, but related back to the energy levels a person may have. Colette has kindly created a diagram to illustrate her own experience with this (Figure 8.1), showing how the impact of a task that drains her of energy can have a knock-on impact on her social and emotional well-being.

Thinking back to Chapter 4, the measurements in complex care included social health as well as mental health outcomes (see Table 4.2); you can see why this is a vital part when we consider the lives of our patients holistically. Multidisciplinary team working helps us with that; including social workers and psychologists provides us with a viewpoint that traditionally considers those aspects. But it illustrates the importance of putting the person at the heart of it; without keeping the focus on the person we are caring for, we forget that their choices should be front and foremost in our minds. Although decision-making can be challenging in some circumstances, the person may be clear on the need they have (Colette's motor in her chair, for example), and focusing on other needs will be not only a waste of energy for all involved but also counterproductive in terms of producing the trust required in this area of practice – think back to

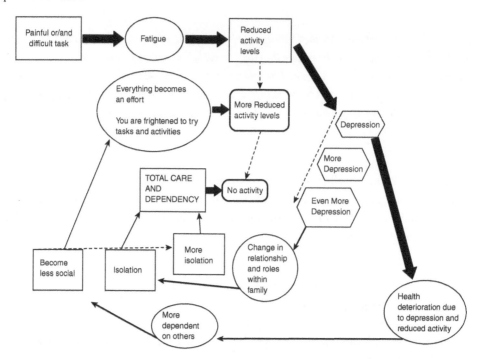

Figure 8.1 Colette's flow chart illustrating downward spiral of a difficult or painful task leading to total dependence and isolation (adapted into black and white), permission signed

Chapter 6, where the IP-SDM Mechanism Map (Figure 6.2) put trust and anxiety in the first stage of decision-making. Without trust, built on an authentic relationship, decision-making for care planning becomes significantly less effective and less useful.

Activity 8.5   Communication

Frequently, a patient referred to the complex care team is working through their own emotions around their situation, diagnosis, or symptoms. How might your communication skills need to be applied in this situation? What skills would you use to ensure the trust was built in the early stages of the relationship and their anxiety alleviated?

A brief outline answer is provided at the end of this chapter.

Sexuality as an activity of daily living

One element of trust and communication is the ability of the professional to discuss topics that are sensitive to the person in a way that is actively not harmful and is compassionate and evidence-based. These sensitive areas may be personal, often based in the trauma we discussed in Chapter 4 (see Figure 4.2), or cultural, such as money, status, or sexuality. Earlier, we have discussed the Roper–Logan–Tierney model; note the sexual element of that now. This is a frequently ignored area of care and one where the impact is underestimated. This is not only the case for adults with disabilities but with older people as well. McGrath et al. (2021) demonstrate, in their quality systematic mixed methods review, that the primary barriers are in fact the healthcare professionals – only 14.2 per cent routinely asked about sexuality or provided patients with information around it. The patient is highly unlikely to raise the topic themselves, but even when they do, the skill of the healthcare professional may make the situation awkward and something to be avoided, so sexual function remains a taboo topic. You can see the impact of that awkwardness in the case of Binita.

Case study: Binita

Binita is a young woman with early-onset Parkinson's; dating is an issue for her. Her mobility is currently at a stage where she can walk independently; she still experiences periods where the medication wears off and her function drops radically (known as wearing off). She approaches her specialist nurse to discuss her options for managing this, stating it is impacting on her sex life. Her specialist nurse clearly is uncomfortable with the conversation, brushing over it and suggesting that it is something that is unimportant compared to the other symptoms under discussion (urinary issues and pain management).

Activity 8.6   Evidence-based practice and research

When thinking about the scenario above, what might you consider suggesting the nurse read? Is her practice evidence-based or is it based on her own beliefs about Binita's situation?

Seek out one quality journal article to support evidence-based practice around disability and sexuality and compare it to the nurse's practice.

As this activity is based on your own thoughts, no outline answer is provided at the end of the chapter.

One of the reasons this interaction may have been so awkward and uncomfortable was the lack of training the healthcare worker received around sexual health; Gerbild et al. (2018) found that a short course changed the attitudes of students, removing the barriers to the conversations about sexual health. Abwao et al. (2021) found that sexuality for people with disabilities was viewed through medical, financial and gendered lenses, where everyone had opinions on spending government money to support someone in expressing their sexuality; that males were viewed differently from other genders; and that people felt they had the right to discuss the reproductive choices of people with disabilities. When we consider that this is the context of the conversation in the scenario, we can see the increased barriers and anxieties around it. We can see the potential consequences in Bettie's statement below.

Case study: Bettie

This statement may be triggering to those with a history of sexual abuse. Please feel free to move on if you feel it may be difficult for you to read.

In her own words:

As a survivor/victim of childhood sexual abuse my sexual health has proved to be an incredibly difficult but nevertheless important issue. It has been systematically ignored by a succession of healthcare practitioners, whether they be nurses, doctors or psychologists. It is recorded in my notes several times that I was suffering with difficulties with intimacy, but no-one has ever suggested psychosexual counselling to address my problems. I am more than aware of the issues I have and so is my husband. I am more than aware of how those problems have affected my marriage and in turn my mental health – and probably my husband's too. But nobody, not one single person, has suggested any help – and that is because no-one ever asks about my sexual health. It has now been over twenty years since I was last intimate in any way with my husband – too late for it to be rectified. I feel that the system has failed me – and my husband come to that, because they were too scared to start that conversation with me. Yes, I was abused. Yes, it was traumatic and, yes, I am still suffering the aftereffects but surely that is what makes me a person with complex needs?

Even our own NMC requirements do not address sexuality in the same way as other ADLs; it positions sexual behaviours as something that impacts mental, physical and behavioural health and well-being, in the same area as smoking, substance and alcohol use (NMC Platform 2.4). It does list other ADLs we should use evidence-based care in, such as nutrition, hydration, bladder and bowel health, mobility, hygiene, oral care, wound care and skin integrity (NMC Platform 4.6 and 4.7). But not sexuality.

Simple and yet vital pieces of knowledge are missed because we do not have these conversations and it may illustrate the way we view our patients as asexual beings, rather than whole adults (Abwao et al., 2021) – historically, their sexuality has been policed in a way that other groups have not been. Equally, without opening those conversations, we cannot identify when a patient might be placed in a risky situation – some conditions and medications have side-effects which can be uncomfortable or socially taboo to discuss. Sometimes opening the door to a conversation provides information on a difficult issue, as it does in the case of Binita.

Case study: Binita

Binita returns to her specialist nurse after a medication adjustment – her neurologist has added in a dopamine agonist. When the specialist nurse opens the conversation around that medication, she mentions one of the potential side-effects known as impulse control disorder, where patients may engage in behaviours previously unknown such as increased or new sexual drives, shopping, or gambling. Binita admits that she has been spending more money on impulsive purchases and this has led to financial difficulties.

Mental health and adults with complex needs

In Chapter 7, we discussed the issues raised by living with mental health complex needs and it addressed issues such as capacity and consent, but briefly we want to highlight that depression and anxiety are common for adults with complex needs, and that this may be another sensitive conversation that is necessary to have; earlier in the chapter we spoke of the grief and loss that can be experienced and these concepts are interlinked.

Think back to Bettie (see Chapter 3, Activity 3.1); we spoke about the impact moving from a respected role in society to being judged for claiming benefits made on her well-being and mental health. Recall your reflection from that chapter (Activity 3.3) around the impact of financial stress and loss of income. Although depression and anxiety can rise as a symptom of a particular condition, they are often symptoms of the intersection between our society and culture, and the situation of the person with complex needs. As with the physical, emotional and intellectual budgeting, the pressures we have discussed throughout this book force people with complex needs to make financial and social choices, and all of this has an impact. As soon as you put yourself in a position to see through the lens of their experience, you become a better ally to your patients – understanding the impact of broader, society-level structures allows you to support them in navigating the barriers created by that, just as your understanding of the way the NHS works allows you to help them in that area.

Activity 8.7   Reflection

In what ways can you ensure that you attempt to view the patient's world from their perspective rather than a medical one?

As this activity is based on your own reflection, no outline answer is provided at the end of the chapter.

Chapter summary

The NMC Code places a duty on us to be advocates for our patients at every level of society, from individual to political, and unless we examine our own practice daily, we cannot meet that duty. Throughout this book, we have attempted to show you the multiple ways that social and political determinants of health can influence the care of an individual living with complex needs. In this chapter, we have discussed some specifics to the needs of adults, and illustrated these with individual case studies, both shared by our experts and drawn from experiences in practice.

Activities: brief outline answers

Activity 8.2 Critical thinking (page 124)

It is worth noting that the funding for support animals is often placed on charities. The cost can be up to £30,000, not including the 'puppy parents' who raise the puppy for its first year. The costs of the animal living with the person are still required – so they must find a budget to cover food, insurance and vet bills. It could save a considerable proportion of carer time but is not funded.

Modern technology can help reduce energy drain but again often must be self-funded, where the system does not consider those 'special' or extra items. Understanding what would help is a major barrier – Colette makes the point that occupational therapists have a considerable amount of training to understand what is helpful, but access can be a problem. Providing earlier access may prevent escalation to the next level, but closures of disability living centres have become a barrier.

Flexibility of packages to allow carer time which can perform specific tasks is there but those little, smaller things that occur during the rest of the time often are a drain on energy.

Buying ready-made meals can be helpful but they are often repetitive, expensive and may have increased salt.

Activity 8.3 Team working (page 124)

You might have considered these professionals:

- occupational therapist
- physiotherapists
- wheelchair services
- GP practice nurse
- pain clinic staff.

Colette provided a note on this activity: *what I want is just a normal life, being relatively pain free and being able to go out and about when and where I want.*

Activity 8.4 Critical thinking (page 125)

You might consider:

- guide dogs for sight loss;
- mental health support dogs, e.g., autism, very high stress levels;
- PET dogs who visit care homes, etc. for socialising, calming and so on. They are pets who are outgoing and like to be fussed. There is some training involved, mainly for their owners;
- medical alert dogs for people who collapse without warning; these dogs detect changes in body odour and alert the person to get on the floor – for epilepsy, diabetes, etc.;
- canine partners for physical assistance;
- sometimes a dog is dual trained.

Activity 8.5 Communication (page 126)

Very often what has become 'normal' to the person concerned would not be accepted by the public. Colette offered these suggestions and we have used her words here:

- *it takes time to go through everything and as the talk progresses more and more comes out;*
- *don't make light of the situation because the person seems OK with everything and is not depressed (someone once said that if they were in my position they would be depressed, if that is so then am I going to be depressed for the next 40 years?);*
- *taking notes throughout is good because there will be lots to consider and remember, but copious note taking means you will miss some of the conversation and indicate you are not really listening;*
- *confirming what you have heard by looking at your notes can be reassuring and may even highlight something missed;*
- *try to write up notes afterwards rather than after three other visits at the end of the day.*

Annotated further reading

https://www.health.org.uk/publications/a-practical-guide-to-self-management-support

This page has a considerable amount of information on how self-management can be done well.

https://www.rcn.org.uk/magazines/health-and-care/2018/lets-talk-about-sex

This interview discusses the importance of discussing sex with residents in a care home.

Useful websites

https://www.esaorguk.com/

This page contains a lot of information about support animals.

https://www.patients-association.org.uk/self-management

An organisation that advocates for patients but has useful sources for self-management.

Chapter 9 Complex care in learning disabilities

Sam Greedy and Nick Preddy

NMC Future Nurse: standards of proficiency for registered nurses

Platform 1: Being an accountable professional

1.3 understand and apply the principles of courage, transparency and the professional duty of candour, recognising and reporting any situations, behaviours or errors that could result in poor care outcomes

1.4 demonstrate an understanding of, and the ability to challenge, discriminatory behaviour

1.9 understand the need to base all decisions regarding care and interventions on people's needs and preferences, recognising and addressing any personal and external factors that may unduly influence their decisions

Platform 2: Promoting health and preventing ill health

2.9 use appropriate communication skills and strength based approaches to support and enable people to make informed choices about their care to manage health challenges in order to have satisfying and fulfilling lives within the limitations caused by reduced capability, ill health and disability

2.10 provide information in accessible ways to help people understand and make decisions about their health, life choices, illness and care

Platform 3: Assessing needs and planning care

3.3 demonstrate and apply knowledge of all commonly encountered mental, physical, behavioural and cognitive health conditions, medication usage and treatments when undertaking full and accurate assessments of nursing care needs and when developing, prioritising and reviewing person-centred care plans

3.6 effectively assess a person's capacity to make decisions about their own care and to give or withhold consent

3.7   understand and apply the principles and processes for making reasonable adjustments

3.8   understand and apply the relevant laws about mental capacity for the country in which you are practising when making decisions in relation to people who do not have capacity

Platform 4: Providing and evaluating care

4.1   demonstrate and apply an understanding of what is important to people and how to use this knowledge to ensure their needs for safety, dignity, privacy, comfort and sleep can be met, acting as a role model for others in providing evidence-based person-centred care

4.4   demonstrate the knowledge and skills required to support people with commonly encountered mental health, behavioural, cognitive and learning challenges, and act as a role model for others in providing high quality nursing interventions to meet people's needs

Chapter aims

After reading this chapter you will be able to:

- understand the key characteristics of autistic spectrum conditions
- apply your understanding of those key characteristics to providing individualised, person-centred care sensitive to the needs of individuals with autism
- understand some key concepts in working with people with complex behaviours in a range of environments and settings
- understand the functional aspects of complex behaviour
- apply your understanding to developing effective strategies to support people with complex behaviours.

Introduction

There are approximately 1.5 million people with learning disabilities in the UK (Mencap, 2021), which is approximately 2.16 per cent of the population. The causes of learning disabilities are many and varied, and each person with a diagnosis of a learning disability has a different lived experience of their condition. Additionally, there is wide variation in the complexity of the needs of those individuals, with some people living full, healthy and independent lives, to others with complex co-morbid health needs, mental health conditions, or complex behaviours who require 24-hour care and support. In your practice you will be required to work with people with learning disabilities, and the idea of this chapter is to help you consider some effective ways of doing this. Learning Disabilities Nurses aim to champion the cause of people with learning disabilities, and we would want you to do the same.

Defining learning disabilities

There are various definitions of learning disabilities, with some minor international differences in content and terminology, but since the publication of *Valuing People: A New Strategy for Learning Disability for the 21st Century* (Department of Health, 2001), in the UK the following has been accepted in most cases as a broad definition:

> *Learning Disability includes the presence of:*
>
> - *A significantly reduced ability to understand new or complex information, to learn new skills (impaired intelligence), with;*
> - *A reduced ability to cope independently (impaired social functioning);*
> - *which started before adulthood, with a lasting effect on development.*
>
> (Department of Health, 2001, p. 14)

The definition in *Valuing People* explicitly states that although measuring learning disability by using IQ as a reference point has some merit, it should not be used as the sole indicator (Department of Health, 2001).

There is a debate as to whether defining learning disability at all, is a valuable exercise, or indeed a damaging one. Atherton and Crickmore (2011) argue that learning disabilities is a constructed idea that hangs a label around a person's neck, which may have negative consequences for the person. Adhering to the idea of the *Social Model of Disability* (Scope, 2022), Atherton and Crickmore (2011, p. 6) point out that *You simply cannot be a person with a Learning Disability on your own.*

Activity 9.1   Critical thinking

Consider some of the 'labels' that you have heard applied to people regarding, for example, their ethnicity, colour, sexuality, disability, mental health diagnosis, gender, age, political stance (i.e., 'snowflake').

- What images or stereotypes does this give rise to in your mind (with or without evidence)?
- Consider any labels, positive or negative, that have been applied to you. Are they true?
- What could the negative impact on a person's life be if they are given the 'label' of exhibiting 'challenging behaviour'?

An outline answer is provided at the end of this chapter.

As nurses it is important to be able to empathise with our patients/service users, so we hope that exercise helped you to get inside the experience a little.

Case study: Mark

Commentary in his own words:

Having learning disabilities doesn't mean there is something wrong with me. I just need support with some things, the same as you all do. Like Nick (Preddy) always needs help with technology because he doesn't understand it!

Some diagnosed learning disabilities have some additional health needs associated with them, such as Down's syndrome and dementia, Rhett's syndrome and gastro-intestinal problems and scoliosis in later life (Rodoconachi-Roidi et al., 2018). There is a higher incidence of epilepsy (up to 33 per cent) in people with learning disabilities (Gates et al., 2014), for example, and a range of other chronic conditions caused by lifestyle and issues such as lack of mobility.

In most cases the medical treatment will be the same, but issues of accessibility and support may be different.

Case study: Mark

Commentary in his own words:

When I go to the doctor or dentist, I want people to:

- *listen to me*
- *get to know me*
- *give me enough time*
- *stick to appointment times*
- *have my support worker with me (if I need her)*
- *talk to me first (not my support worker)*
- *use words and language I understand.*

As academics and Learning Disabilities Nurses, the two things that we are asked about most, and cause our colleagues – particularly in Adult Nursing – the most anxiety are:

- autism; and
- complex (or 'challenging') behaviour.

These often cause people with learning disabilities to require residential staff, families, or other carers to support the person in healthcare settings as the staff in the setting find understanding and supporting people with these conditions difficult, stressful and even frightening. We have experience of staff we worked with in a care home being asked by nurses on a hospital ward to administer medication to a person with disabilities while on the hospital ward; the nurses often felt so out of their depth due to the idea of 'challenging behaviour', which we will consider here.

Challenging behaviour

We know that health and social care services are stretched and are frequently working at capacity – and supporting someone with a learning disability and challenging behaviour can take additional time and resources. It can also feel scary, as we can often worry about doing the 'right' thing, particularly when there could be the risk of being hurt. We should aim to understand behaviour and minimise risk. If that is the best thing for our patients or service users and us, shouldn't we do this?

Defining challenging behaviour

Before we define challenging behaviour, we need to consider what 'behaviour' is.

Our behaviour is everything that we do, all our observable actions and movements. We all engage in behaviour.

Box 9.1   Definitions

When we define challenging behaviour, there are three main definitions we can use:

Culturally abnormal behaviour of such an intensity, frequency or duration that the physical safety of the person or others is likely to be placed in serious jeopardy, or behaviour which is likely to limit seriously use of, or result in the person being denied access to, ordinary community facilities.

(Emerson, 1995, p. 3)

Behaviour of such an intensity, frequency or duration as to threaten the quality of life and/or the physical safety of the individual or others and is likely to lead to responses that are restrictive, aversive or result in exclusion.

(Royal College of Psychiatrists, British Psychological Society and Royal College of Speech and Language Therapists, 2007, p. 10)

a problem may be considered to exist if it satisfies at least some of the following criteria:

- *The behaviour itself or its severity is inappropriate given a person's age or level of development*

- *The behaviour is dangerous either to the person or others*

- *The behaviour constitutes a significant additional handicap for the person by interfering with the learning of new skills or by excluding the person from important learning opportunities*

- *The behaviour causes significant stress to those who live and work with the person and impairs the quality of their lives to a significant degree*

- *The behaviour is contrary to social norms.*

(Zarkowska and Clements, 1996, p. 3)

These definitions broadly consider similar criteria to define challenging behaviour. However, behaviour is much more nuanced than these definitions and there are additional considerations that we may need to make.

- *The social rules guarding what constitutes appropriate behaviour in that setting.* Some behaviours are appropriate in a particular context. For example, we should all be spitting at least twice a day, as we brush our teeth. However, if we started spitting on the floor of a café, this would be seen as an inappropriate behaviour. It is also important to consider what is age-appropriate around, for example, continence.
- *The capacity of the setting to manage any disruption caused by the person's behaviour.* We can say that challenging behaviour is any behaviour which challenges the system. This means that the threshold for what is challenging will vary depending on the type of service, the skills of staff and the understanding of what behaviour is.

Activity 9.2   Critical thinking

List as many different types of challenging behaviour as you can think of.

As this activity is based on your own critical thinking, no outline answer is provided at the end of this chapter.

Looking at the list you have made, you should be able to group those behaviours into categories:

- aggression to others (probably the behaviour that we feel most worried about);
- aggression to self – self-injurious behaviours. This can often be challenging to observe and can be upsetting, particularly if someone has hurt themselves;
- aggression to the environment – such as damage to property;
- socially inappropriate behaviours – this may be behaviours such as shouting, removing clothes or masturbation in public;
- stereotypies – these are repetitive behaviours which someone might engage in. For example, if someone is asking the same question again and again, this may feel very challenging to manage.

These behaviours are very complex, so why do they happen?

The functions of behaviour

When we speak to staff teams or families about the behaviours which they are finding challenging, the biggest question is always *but why is it happening?* It is easy to feel that there is absolutely no reason for a behaviour. It is important to remember that behaviour is about communication – communicating what someone wants or doesn't want. There is always a reason for behaviour.

There are four main functions for behaviour:

1. wanting something (i.e., food or objects);
2. avoidance (i.e., activities, people, or objects);
3. wanting attention;
4. sensory stimulation, which may mean engaging in a behaviour because you like the sensation that it gives.

Some people add a fifth function: communicating a pain or feeling unwell.

As nurses, sometimes we need to be detectives, and we need to work out what the function of someone's behaviour is. Using behaviour-recording charts like ABC charts can help us by recording what happened before an incident (the Antecedent), what happened during the incident (the Behaviour) and what happened after (the Consequence). This can give us some more information about the behaviour, particularly where the reason why does not seem clear. The more information we can include on these, the better we can understand the behaviour, and use this to inform our behaviour management and care plans.

So why are people with a learning disability likely to present with behaviours which we find challenging? We have thought about how behaviour is linked to communication and communicating an unmet need. If someone finds it more difficult to communicate verbally, they are more likely to use their behaviour to tell us what they need. We often respond more quickly to behaviour, particularly if someone is hurting themselves or is hurting someone else. This makes the behaviour very effective and is a motivation to continue to engage in that behaviour.

A note on physical health

Remember that someone may have an underlying health concern or pain which is contributing towards their behaviour. A person's physical health should be one of the first things that we look at, to rule out a condition which we could treat or manage. Some common conditions to explore include:

- ear infections
- urinary tract infections
- constipation/bowel problems
- epilepsy
- dental problems
- eyesight
- pica (consider if someone has swallowed something inedible)
- side effects of medication
- sleep issues
- diet issues.

There is a risk of diagnostic overshadowing where the *symptoms of physical ill health are mistakenly attributed to either a mental health/behavioural problem or as being inherent in the person's learning disabilities* (Emerson and Baines, 2010, p. 9). We should see any change in a person's behaviour as a potential sign of ill health, until we have ruled this out.

The Time-Intensity model (Kaplan and Wheeler, 1983)

The Time-Intensity model or escalation curve describes the different stages someone may go through when they become overstimulated, or agitation begins to increase to the point of crisis. My team represented this in pictorial form, as an anger volcano (Figure 9.1).

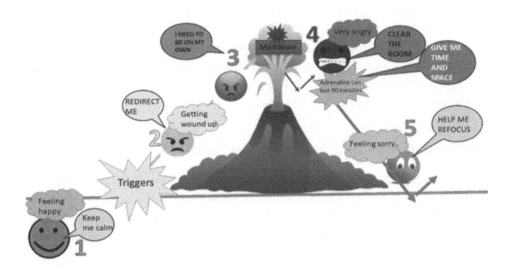

Figure 9.1 Anger volcano

Baseline

This is where someone is calm and settled – and where we want our patients and service users to stay. At this level of arousal, people are most able to communicate and engage with us. Everyone's baseline is different, but it is the time when people are most likely to engage. This may be affected by the person's learning disability. At this stage, we can use proactive strategies to keep someone calm.

Triggers and escalation

A trigger is something which we perceive to be a threat. This may be something which is observable, or this may be unobservable, such as an internal trigger or a memory. We may not always know what the trigger is, or it may have occurred a while ago. Once a trigger has occurred, a person will begin to escalate. For some people, this will be slow. In others, this could be very quick. We can use redirection or distraction here to prevent a crisis occurring.

Crisis

Some people call this stage 'meltdown'. In a crisis, the priority is safety management. Keep yourself and others safe. Don't feel like you are not doing enough. In an incident, we feel like we need to be in control by doing something. Immediately after an incident, make sure that you do not return to them straight away. Someone may be retriggered which may lead to another crisis immediately after, as they may not have had time to return to baseline.

Post-incident

After an incident, we may see a 'dip', where someone becomes withdrawn or tired. Consider what someone might need. Do they need some space before you support them? Do they need an activity to distract them? Do they need any first aid? There is often the temptation to dive in and try and analyse what happened and debrief with the person, but this may not be the most helpful thing to do. There may be consequences after an incident, such as someone not being able to engage in an activity, or not having an object because it has been broken. However, we need to make sure that we are not punishing people after an incident.

Remembering self-care and management

As nurses supporting people who may present with behaviour which is more challenging at times, it is important that we look after ourselves. Make sure you consider your own self-management strategies to avoid your own crisis. This is not the time to be a hero. If you need time and space, make sure you utilise this. After an incident, make sure you use debrief and supervision for support.

Activity 9.3   Reflection

- What do you need at each stage of the escalation curve?
- What keeps you at baseline?
- What do you need if there is a trigger?
- What do you need to avoid reaching crisis?
- What do you need when you reach crisis?
- What do you need after an incident?

As this activity is based on your own reflection, no outline answer is provided at the end of this chapter.

To summarise this section:

- all behaviour is a form of communication;
- we need to understand what the function of the behaviour is and meet that need;
- we need to make sure we look after ourselves and reflect as we support people who are engaging in behaviours we might find challenging.

Activity 9.4 Reflection

If you have worked in a healthcare service, you may have experienced a person with learning disabilities accessing your service. What support did they have when they accessed your service?

What might the challenges be in supporting the person effectively?

An outline answer is provided at the end of this chapter.

Arguably, this lack of knowledge and understanding of people with learning disabilities and their needs has led to significant health inequalities highlighted in the *Confidential Inquiry into Premature Deaths of People with Learning Disabilities* (Norah Fry Research Centre, 2013) and the *Death by Indifference* report (Mencap, 2007), both of which evidence institutionalised discrimination in healthcare services.

In this chapter we will explore the two issues mentioned above (autism and complex behaviours). They are, of course, just two issues among many, but the basic principles of good assessment, appropriate treatment, flexibility of service provision and valuing people with learning disabilities, complex needs and autism as equal members of society with equal rights to good healthcare discussed in this chapter can be applied in most situations.

Understanding autism

Before proceeding to a definition and description of key elements of autism, it is worth noting that autism is an umbrella phrase for a range of presentations that are uniquely individual to each person who has this label. Described as a 'spectrum' condition (National Autistic Society, 2021), this means that it encompasses a wide range of ways that each individual experiences and processes the world. Although here we must speak in generalisations, no two people with autism are the same.

Just a note on terminology and 'person-first' language. In a recent conversation with an autistic person, she asked me to use 'autistic person', so here that will be used. This is supported by the National Autistic Society.

Interestingly, autistic people are beginning to appear with more regularity in popular culture. Slightly controversially, Ricky Gervais portrayed an autistic person in his sitcom *Derek*, Benedict Cumberbatch has played Sherlock Holmes by emphasising recognisable traits such as difficulties with social interaction, heightened senses and an eye for detail and the most recognisable is probably Sheldon Cooper as played by Jim Parsons in *The Big Bang Theory*.

Most of these characters are played sympathetically with strengths and positives identified and celebrated as much as the many struggles that each character experiences.

Definition

Both the DSM-5 and ICD-10 categorisations of autism include two main elements (National Autistic Society, 2021):

- persistent difficulties with social interaction and communication; and
- a range of restricted and repetitive interests and patterns of behaviour (including sensory processing).

These have been present since early childhood and are lifelong.

Before we go further into this topic, we would ask you to consider a commonly held view, and statement that we hear quite regularly: *Everyone is a little bit on the autistic spectrum.* Although the neuro-typical may empathise, we think this statement somewhat cheapens and trivialises the everyday lived experience of autistic people. Please read this chapter and form your own view.

Diagnosis and incidence

According to the National Autistic Society (2021), one in every hundred people in the UK is autistic. Diagnosis rates across the world vary, but recent years have seen a sharp rise in the number of diagnoses. In a recent study (Russel et al., 2021), a 787 per cent increase in diagnoses was recognised between 1998 and 2018. They conclude that this is predominantly due to increased reporting and recognition rather than a significant rise in incidence. A gender bias towards males has been recognised and the National Autistic Society (2021) put a current figure on this as 3:1, although they recognise that research has shown a variety of ratios. Reasons for this are debated and range from biological causes to social causes (Mandy and Lai, 2017).

Diagnosis would generally be undertaken by a psychologist following a referral via GP (adult) or teacher (child), although more people are self-referring for private assessments (Russel et al., 2021). Waiting times for diagnosis can be very long, and this has been identified as an issue by the government in the latest *National Strategy* (Department of Health and Social Care, 2021a).

Causes

Current thinking is away from psychological causes, and strongly towards the idea of genetic causes. This is now supported by much of the science (Casanova and Casanova, 2019; Rylaarsdam and Guemez-Gamboa, 2019) and investigation into this element is continuing.

Rylaarsdam and Guemez-Gamboa (2019) conclude that the genetic element to the causation of autism was recognised by the early 2000s with reference to a range of research, including studies of twins showing high concordance in monozygotic twins and a strong relation between the amount of genetic material shared with parents and siblings who are affected by autism. No single specific cause or gene has been identified (Fletcher-Watson and Happé, 2019) and the likelihood is that there are many different genetic causes, specific to each autistic person. This individuality is one of the most baffling, but wonderful elements of the condition.

There is evidence that vaccines do not cause autism, but there is likely to be an environmental element such as maternal illnesses like diabetes and thyroid disease, prematurity, parental age and exposure to some medications (Casanova and Casanova, 2019; Hodges et al., 2020). Foetal exposure to valproic acid (used in some anti-epileptic drugs) is indicated (Casanova and Casanova, 2019; Hodges et al., 2020; Rylaarsdam and Guemez-Gamboa, 2019). The research into causes of autism continues.

Social interaction

Baron-Cohen et al. (2009) recognise the processing problems that autistic people experience that cause issues such as recognising emotional states of others from body language, verbal language, voice intonations and facial expressions. Frith (2008) considers that the complexity of social interaction and the variety of voices, sounds, faces (eyes, mouth, etc.) and body language make it harder for people to process and interpret information.

Literal understanding and use of language

The National Autistic Society (2021) points out that autistic people may tend to take things a person says literally, and not to understand the more abstract and social elements of language. Frith (1989) gives an example where she is at the dinner table with an autistic person and asks the person if they can pass the salt, to which the person replies 'Yes', but does not pass the salt, missing the social and practical element of the question. In a literal sense, this is the correct answer.

Socially, there are many mutually agreed meanings of words and phrases. The use of sarcasm and 'banter' are examples of these. Sheldon Cooper struggles with sarcasm in particular in the early stages of *The Big Bang Theory* TV series, relying on his companions to tell him when people are being sarcastic.

Activity 9.5   Critical thinking

Think of and write down five sayings and 'idioms' that we use regularly that could confuse an autistic person, and which you might want to avoid when interacting with them.

An outline answer is provided at the end of this chapter.

There can be a correlating use of very direct and literal language, such as criticising a person's appearance. A potential cause of this is a difficulty in understanding other people's emotions and sensitivity to social cues and body language (Baron-Cohen et al., 2009). This can lead to people seeming insensitive and tactless and becomes a barrier to developing friendships and relationships.

There can also be a very formal use of words and phrases, and the need to fully articulate a topic regardless of the interest of the listener (Attwood, 2007). We have experienced a person who used 'incorrect' but literal pronouns when singing along to a song, where 'I can't get you out my head' (from the Kylie Minogue song) becomes 'she can't get him out of her head'. This idiosyncratic language can also be a barrier to relationships.

The importance of eye contact in developing relationships is well reported (Stickley, 2011), but it can be very difficult for autistic people (Williams, 2006; Bogdashina, 2003) – for example, even avoiding watching the eyes of people on screen. Frith (2008) cites research showing that people may watch chins rather than eyes. Research by Jones and Klin (2013) shows a decline in 'eye looking' in babies later diagnosed with autism between two and six months of age.

These things have led people to think that autistic people do not want to have interaction, but the more we read from people like Donna Williams and Willow Hope we see that people do (on the whole) want friendships and relationships, but just find it harder than neuro-typical people. In her book *The Girl in the Panda Hat* (2012), Willow Hope published several poems highlighting this:

'I'm Just Invisible Me'

What's it going to take for you to see?

This whole thing seems such a waste,

Well would you even notice me?

If I weren't screaming into your face.

Being alone hurts the most,

When you're also so alone.

I sometimes feel like a ghost,

Walking into the unknown,

I know you don't see me,

And I know I don't exist,

I know that I'm lucky,

Therefore I won't be missed,

I wish just once you'd look my way,

Then maybe you might see,

And listen to what I have to say,

But of course not – I'm just invisible me.

Most of us in our lives have had some experience of loneliness and isolation, and I urge you to consider these things when interacting with autistic people who may be at greater risk.

Restricted and repetitive interests and patterns of behaviour

The National Autistic Society (2021) points out that for autistic people the world can appear an overwhelming and confusing place. There are a multitude of sensory and emotional experiences happening all the time.

The restricted and repetitive interests and patterns of behaviours are often the autistic person's way of managing this situation by imposing some sort of order upon a difficult and disordered world.

Behaviours can include:

- rocking
- spinning
- hand movements ('flapping')
- vocalisations
- manipulating objects with hands and fingers (beads, string, rough objects, soft objects, hard objects)
- repeated movements (walking the same short pattern of steps)
- a focus on specific topics, often talking in great detail
- repeated routines (such as arranging toys in certain way, repeated routes to destinations, etc)
- only eating food of certain textures of colours, or having them arranged in a certain way on a plate
- only wearing specific clothes, or having very strong favourite clothing, shoes, duvet cover, curtains, etc.
- a general reliance on things remaining the same.

Previously seen as negative 'obsessions', there is an extraordinary video by autistic blogger Amanda Baggs called *In My Language* (2007) that explores beautifully the depth of interaction an autistic person can be having with their environment as a means of both understanding and engaging with it, even if we find this difficult to interpret in the neuro-typical world (see useful links later in this chapter for details). It shows how behaviours that might be seen as maladaptive or 'obsessions' are in fact part of a unique and deeply treasured interaction with the world, rather than distancing from it.

However positive we intend to be, this behaviour can become an issue for the person and those around them in certain circumstances. When certain rituals must be completed to the exclusion of all other activities the consequences for the person can be difficult to overcome and manage. Autistic people themselves refer to these responses to stressful situations as 'meltdowns' – when the person becomes so overwhelmed by a situation that this may manifest itself as a loss of control of their behaviour either verbally or physically and that they can be misconstrued as tantrums, especially in children (National Autistic Society, 2021). They cite the possibility of a 'shutdown', which is a quieter, more introverted way of the person dealing with the situation, where they may go very quiet, or immobile, unable to move until they have processed the situation and been able to react.

It is important when working and interacting with autistic people that we are aware of the triggers that this individual may experience, and how they can be affected by the environment, and inevitable disruptions to those routines and rituals. Our own behaviour and how we manage the environment around an autistic person may have a profound effect on how effective our healthcare interventions, even unexpected ones can be.

Sensory issues

In this next section we are going to explore some basic sensory issues that autistic people can experience, caused by their differences in sensory processing. They are extremely important for professionals working with autistic people, as working proactively to manage the environment around an autistic person may be one of the most effective and sensitive ways that we can support a person. A little awareness and sensitivity can go a long way.

Bogdashina (2003) explores perceptual issues for autistic people and considers seven sensory systems, or senses, including the five we traditionally identify:

- visual (sight)
- tactile (touch)
- auditory (hearing)
- olfactory (smell)
- gustation (taste).

And two further senses: the vestibular and proprioceptive systems.

The vestibular system is how elements such as balance, judgement of distance, depth perception and head positioning are processed via the inner ear and visual cortex; the proprioceptive system senses how the body occupies space, proximity and generally how the person is placed in the world.

For the purposes of this chapter, we are going to focus more on touch, hearing, smell, taste and sight. There are specific therapies that trained professionals might use to support a person over the long term to help them learn how to better understand and process the world more effectively regarding the vestibular and proprioceptive systems. Sensory integration therapy has been an essential part of occupational therapists' work with people with sensory processing issues since Ayres' study in the 1970s (May-Benson and Schaaf, 2014; Soderback, 2014).

Hyper- and hyposensitivity

Broadly, autistic people's experiences of sensory stimuli fall into two categories 'hyper-sensitivity' and 'hyposensitivity'. This is something of an over-simplification, but when experiencing stimuli in a 'hypersensitive' way the autistic person may experience the stimulus very strongly, whether than be a sound, a sight, an aroma, a taste, or the experience of physical contact, and when experiencing stimuli in a 'hyposensitive way' the experience can be muted or nonexistent.

In hypersensitivity it may be a multitude of those experiences which the person cannot switch off or filter out and may cause 'sensory overload'. Neuro-typical people mostly can be aware of but filter out peripheral sounds and sights and focus (naturally) on the specific stimuli that are important at that time. They are able to 'switch channels' and focus on something else if prompted to do so, which you may be able to do if you consciously now think of moving your attention away from this book (using your eyes) to other senses that you have been aware of and processing but ignoring until you have to pay attention.

Sensory overload can be very challenging for an autistic person, making certain environments very difficult for people to manage, engage with and even remain in. This may be an overload of too many sounds, or smells, or visual stimuli, or physical stimuli, or tastes individually, or it could be a combination of some or all of those types of stimuli.

Hyposensitivity	Possible activity
Sound	• Be attracted to loud noises
	• Make loud noises (verbal such as repeated sounds, or loud shouts and screams)
	• Make loud noises (physically such as banging things or surfaces, shaking things that rattle, etc.)
	• Placing ears close to noises and listening intently
	• Placing hands over ears or potentially banging ears to cause sensation
Tactile experiences	• Rocking and swaying
	• Stamping (for both sound and tactile experience)
	• Attracted to rough surfaces
	• Liking firm pressure on skin and body
	• Playing with brushes, knobbly or rough surfaces and objects
	• Running things through fingers (stones, sand, beads)
	• Banging head against objects
	• Self-injury

(Continued)

Table 9.1 (Continued)

Hyposensitivity	Possible activity
Taste	• Liking very strong-tasting or spicy food and drink
	• Using taste as a way of exploring and experiencing the world
	• Tasting things that are unusual (perhaps dangerous for people to eat)
Smell	• Being attracted to things that smell strongly
	• Liking strong-smelling foods and drinks
	• Using smell as a way of exploring and experiencing the world
Vision	• Being attracted to and interested in bright or flashing/twinkling lights
	• Getting close to lights, TV, etc.
	• Manipulating light to make a more distinctive experience (i.e., waving objects or fingers in a shaft of sunlight to disturb it)
	• Watching and following things that wave or flap (flags, things on a washing line, etc.)

Table 9.1 Hyposensitivities

The need to recognise each autistic person's individuality and support needs regarding this is worth restating here.

Activity 9.6   Critical thinking

Consider your work environment for a moment and make a list of all the different sensory experiences that someone might have in that work environment, either as someone who works there (you may have a colleague who is autistic) or as a patient/service user.

List all the noises, smells, tastes, tactile experiences, visual experiences that a person may have.

When you have listed them, consider the following:

• What must it be like (for example) to hear all those sounds very loudly and to not be able to filter any out?
• What must it be like (for example) to experience all the visual stimuli very strongly and to not be able to filter any out?
• What about sounds and visual stimuli together?
• What about all the sensory experiences at once?
• How do you think that you would cope with experiences like that?
• What would help you to be able to manage it?
• What could you do in your workplace to support an autistic person who is experiencing the environment in this way?

The answers to the questions above will be specific and personal to your service, or where you have undertaken practice placements as a student nurse, and you will have been asked to consider your own coping strategies which will be different for each reader.

An outline answer is provided at the end of this chapter.

Although hypersensitivity can present challenges for a person, there can be benefits. We have already mentioned Cumberbatch's portrayal of Sherlock Holmes with heightened senses, ability to remember detail and the ability to see patterns and connections where others cannot. These abilities (to a greater or lesser extent) are a reality for some autistic people and it only takes a small change of attitude to see this as an ability rather than a disability.

It is sometimes reported that high-functioning autistic people are actively recruited for roles in locations such as the Government Communications Head Quarters and, although we suspect this is something of an urban myth, there is no doubt that some of the skills and attributes we have considered above might very well equip someone well to do certain jobs that require focus, concentration, an eye for detail and the ability to spot patterns.

On the other side of the hypersensitivity 'coin' some autistic people experience hyposensitivity, where their sensory experiences in some or all of those areas are muted, and rather than experience exceptionally high levels of sensory input, they experience very little.

A person who is hyposensitive may try to seek out sensory experiences as a way of engaging with the world and people around them. These behaviours may include seeking out strong sensory experiences via touch, smell, sight, sound and taste:

- loud noises (listening and making)
- firm touch, rough surfaces
- rocking/swaying/stamping
- strong-smelling and -tasting food and substances.

This is by no means an exhaustive list and each person will be very different.

Visual and auditory experiences

There are a wide range of visual experiences that autistic people report. Donna Williams (2006) speaks of a range of things that affected her and, although each person experiences different things, there are some common things that people talk about.

- Images fracture, distort and split up, so that they no longer appear whole, or look like they did before.
- Images swim in and out of focus.
- Things far away appear close, and things close appear far away, and these can change and alternate.
- Patterned materials (curtains/carpets) can make an autistic person feel unwell, causing headaches and feelings of nausea.
- Things can be seen in minute overwhelming detail and sharpness.
- Due to the sharpness and intensity of the images eye contact can be uncomfortable and even painful.

As you can imagine, these visual experiences may make for a confusing and disorientating world that lacks the coherence experienced by neuro-typical people.

Auditory experiences

Bogdashina (2003) identifies a similar range of issues that affect autistic people across all areas of sensory perception; auditory experiences are similar to the list above for visual experiences. Such as:

- fragmentation and distortion
- faraway sounds may sound near and vice versa
- difficulty distinguishing between and filtering sounds, particularly in busy environments with multiple sounds
- everything is amplified.

Tactile experiences

There is again a vast range of ways that autistic people experience touch and physical contact, and each person is, of course, different. Below are some commonly reported issues with 'hypertactility' or being hypersensitive to touch.

- Certain fabrics may be uncomfortable.
- Tight clothes or tightness around wrists and throat may be uncomfortable.
- The touch of clothes on any part of their body may be very uncomfortable and be felt as pain for people who are very hypertactile.
- Touch from another person may be uncomfortable.
- Light touch (i.e., brushing against something) may feel worse than firm touch (Heath, in Bradley et al., 2019).

Interventions using firm pressure can be supportive here.

Activity 9.7 Critical thinking

Stop to think for a moment about all the tactile experiences you are having right now all over your body:

- now think of a time when you have had a label sticking into you from clothing, or shoes rubbing, or a collar/tie that was too tight;
- imagine that (or worse), all over your body, all the time; or
- imagine one or two of those things causing you extreme pain or discomfort.

How would that make you feel both physically and emotionally? Please make a list of those feelings.

Now consider your working environment.

- If an autistic person who experiences tactile hypersensitivity were to come into your service how many times, and by what and whom would they be touched?
- How can you lessen the impact of this for an autistic person entering and using your service?

An outline answer is provided at the end of this chapter.

Taste and smell

We have already explored in this chapter how a person who is HYPOsensitive to taste may seek out strong tastes and may need food to be strong in flavour or aroma to get some tangible experience from food and drink. A HYPERsensitive person may find the tastes and smells of food, people, objects, places very strong and overwhelming, and difficult to tolerate (Bogdashina, 2003).

In a previous exercise you were asked to consider the range of smells and other sensory stimuli that can be found in your working place. Please review these now.

In the normal conducting of our work, we may not have to consider these things much unless a person openly expresses a particular dislike, or an allergy, but they are important considerations when working with an autistic person; what we do may either make the experience a bearable, or an unbearable one for our patient/service user.

Final thoughts on sensory issues

When working in a healthcare environment, managing the sensory environment for an autistic person will be an essential part of any care plan, or care given to that person.

It is difficult to capture every issue in a chapter like this, so it is important to emphasise the absolute individuality of each person, the general 'spiky-ness' and variability of autistic people's sensory profiles which can make it difficult to predict. Therefore, we cannot always rely on previous information and assumptions about the person and how they may react.

Co-morbidities

A co-morbidity is where one (or more) additional condition with distinct symptoms from the primary diagnosis is present at the same time, in this case alongside autism (Al-Beltagi, 2021; Casanova et al., 2020).

Space prevents us from exploring these in detail, so what follows is a list of the most common co-morbidities. Getting to know our patients and service users is really important, and your own exploration of how they may potentially affect the autistic person is essential.

- *Learning disabilities*: links to Fragile X and Down's syndromes
- *Neurological conditions*: epilepsy (up to 30 per cent), cerebral palsy, macrocephaly, migraines
- *Gastro-intestinal disorders*: constipation, diarrhoea, reflux, inflammation
- *Sleep disorders*: possibly caused by other issues such as hypersensitivty and other co-morbidities
- *Allergies and auto-immune conditions:* including; asthma, coeliac's disease, type 1 diabetes and rheumatoid arthritis
- *Attention deficit hyperactivity disorder (ADHD), anxiety and other mental health conditions*

It is important for healthcare workers to get to know their individual patients well to be aware of any issues that may arise.

Therapies

In this section we are going to consider a couple of therapies that are commonly used when working with autistic people. Please note that these interventions are not 'cures' for autism, nor are they intended to be 'cures'. Autism and learning disabilities are not diseases, and neither can be, nor need to be cured.

The two interventions considered below (intensive interaction and sensory integration therapy) have a growing and developing evidence base, but practitioners need experience and training to practise these techniques; this chapter does not equip you to do that.

Intensive interaction

Generally spearheaded and championed by Caldwell, an occupational therapist, intensive interaction (II) is a way of communicating with people who are non-verbal by tuning into, and using their own sounds, communication methods and emotional engagement (Bradley et al., 2019). Some of its ideas are based upon the initial communication and relationship building that usually occurs between a baby and its mother in early infancy (Bradley et al., 2019).

The practitioner engaging in II with an autistic person will take account of the sensory needs of the person and try to create an environment as conducive to the person's needs as possible to try to eliminate external factors and make it easier to communicate and engage. The practitioner observes the person for some time to be able to see and get to know and recognise a range of things including vocalisations, sensory experiences, breathing patterns, interactions with environment, movement and emotional reactions.

Only when the observation has taken place and sufficient understanding of the person is held, the practitioner will then start to engage with the person. They will do this by starting to copy and echo back some of the sounds, movements, breathing much in the way that a parent might do with an infant to make an initial engagement. Gurney (in Bradley et al., 2019) describes this as showing the person that they have been recognised and valued and puts aside the apparent meaninglessness (to us) of a behaviour and seeing that it has value to the person.

As the person recognises their own sounds, behaviours and patterns of breathing and movement, the interaction and responses can grow and develop, and a strong relationship can grow. Gurney (2019) and Bradley et al. (2019) cite evidence of the effectiveness of these interactions.

Activity 9.8   Critical thinking

How would you feel about copying and repeating back non-verbal sounds to an adult, or mimicking their movements and breathing?

These interactions may be seen as not being age-appropriate; does this matter?

An outline answer is provided at the end of this chapter.

Sensory integration therapy

Sensory integration therapy (SIT) would generally be led by or undertaken under the supervision of an occupational therapist.

Earlier in this chapter we considered some of the sensory processing issues that autistic people experience. SIT intends to use an assessment of an individual's issues with tactility (touch), proprioception (occupying space, proximity, etc.) and vestibular processing (balance, depth perception, etc.) to support them to manage this effectively and develop skills and improved sensory integration across all senses.

The basic concept is to gently introduce a specifically designed 'diet' of sensory experiences to the person to help them develop their processing and understanding of sensory data (Bogdashina, 2003). Examples of this might be the use of swings and equipment to promote balance such as beams, soft play areas and the like. These activities stimulate the tactile, vestibular and proprioceptive systems in a fun and interactive way, promoting positive communication, socialisation and engagement.

Some more simple strategies that you can use

Below is a list of relatively simple strategies that you could consider in your practice. You can find more information on any of these strategies and resources with a simple internet search.

- *Social stories* are a simple way of helping an autistic person understand and play out a scenario in a simple visual way. They are effectively a comic strip portrayal of a situation, such as attending the GP.
- *Now and next*: a 'now and next' page or book is a simple representation (often visual) of the sequence of activities happening for that person promoting structure and sequence.
- *Picture exchange communication system (PECS)*: working broadly in a similar way to 'now and next' (and possibly in conjunction with it), this is a simple system where the person has a small library of pictures or symbols (or a combination) of key items that they exchange for the real thing, promoting control and communication.
- *Visual timetables*: autistic people often find simple visual representations of something like a timetable (school or personal diary) useful as it helps them picture and visualise the sequence of events, either daily, or over a longer period of time. This can provide a simple guide to expectations and activities.
- *Autism-friendly environment*: a recent development has seen services and shops using quiet periods for visits, longer appointments, subdued lighting and the like. All of these should be individualised and tailored to the person's individual needs. These can also include visual directions and muted sensory experiences.
- *Noise-cancelling headphones/ear defenders*: these help people who have hypersensitive hearing, and can range from ear defenders, which are used to block out as much noise as possible (soundproof), to more sophisticated 'noise-cancelling' headphones.
- *Weighted blankets and clothes*: a weighted blanket is simply what it sounds to be – a blanket or duvet that is filled with weighted material to make it heavier than a normal blanket, thus providing the person with an enhanced or strengthened sensory experience over a significant proportion of their body. It may be possible to have some low-cost items in your workplace.

Perhaps the real key issue here, and what we hope you take away from this chapter, is that we really need to think about our attitude and values regarding people with both learning disabilities and autism. Do we celebrate difference and uniqueness and do whatever it takes to accommodate and support people, or do we fall back on the tired tropes of 'We don't have the time', 'We don't have the money' and 'We don't have the expertise'?

The final exercise asks you to consider how you could make a visit to a hospital ward for an autistic young man (Billy) successful, but the basic principles could be applied in any healthcare, education, or social environment, including your own.

Scenario: Billy

You are a nurse working on a busy twenty-bedded medical ward. In one month, Billy, a sixteen-year-old autistic young man will be spending four days on your ward for a planned medical intervention. Billy has a mild learning disability and communicates verbally with simple three- to four-word sentences. Billy lives at home with his parents, John and Paula, and his older brother James, who is seventeen.

Billy has had a diagnosis of autism and mild learning disabilities since the age of four, although his parents started to suspect that he had a developmental delay when he was as young as eighteen months old.

Billy is very resistant to change and has a visual schedule detailing his activities on each day (including an activity that involves arranging a range of Harry Potter toys in his room, and recreating scenes from the films) and works well with a 'now and next' book. He does not like to meet new people and takes time to get used to them. He responds well to visual tools to understand things. When Billy's routine is changed, he can become very upset and can self-injure by biting his hand. He takes some time to get used to the change. When going to a new place he will walk rapidly up and down the room, will flap his hands and will every now and then scream or swear loudly. He is not always aware of his physical space and can crash into things.

Billy is very sensitive to sensory stimuli. He is hypersensitive to bright colours, busy patterns in curtains and carpets, and he is hypersensitive to sounds and smells, although he likes the smell of one specific Glade plug-in air freshener. If he is in an environment that is too noisy (or with a multitude of sounds), too bright or has strong smells he may experience 'sensory overload' which may lead to a 'meltdown' (crying, screaming and hitting out).

He is particularly sensitive to multiple people speaking around him. Billy is hypersensitive to touch and will only tolerate hugs from his immediate family. Billy has a weighted blanket that he uses at night and also during the day if he is stressed and needs some reassurance. He is very sensitive to certain fabrics and will only wear very specific soft fabrics and colours (mainly pale green). He always sleeps with a Harry Potter duvet (weighted) and pillowcase set. His family has two identical ones that they alternate.

Billy will eat food of all textures safely, but will not eat orange or yellow food, or food that has touched anything else on his plate. Billy is fully mobile and likes to move around freely, but due to his sensory processing difficulties he is not always aware of space around him and can bump into things.

(Continued)

(Continued)

Billy has a very high interest in the Harry Potter films and will talk in detail and at great length about aspects of the films and characters. He becomes very upset if he is not able to finish his monologue about the characters. Billy will interrupt other people to tell them about Harry Potter.

Billy can make simple decisions for himself, but they are based on his own very strict criteria. He considers the advice of his family (especially his mother and brother) to be very important.

Billy's family work with a children's community Learning Disabilities Nurse called Louise who has a very positive relationship with Billy and his family.

Activity 9.9   Critical thinking

How could you work with Billy, his family and other professionals to help Billy manage his stay on your ward and have the medical procedure?

Consider the following.

- Who are the key people to work with and why?
- What might you do before the date of the admission?
- How would you use staff during (and before) the admission?
- How might you adjust the environment to suit Billy?
- What strategies might you use incorporating Billy's interests, and how might these help Billy and you?
- What training and support may staff need?
- Who might you need to liaise with in the hospital and why?

An outline answer is provided at the end of this chapter.

Chapter summary

In this chapter you have learnt about:

- a definition of learning disabilities
- the main characteristics of autism
- the causes of autism
- some simple strategies for supporting autistic people
- understanding the function of 'challenging behaviour'
- the views of people with learning disabilities and autistic people.

Activities: brief outline answers

Activity 9.1 Critical thinking (page 134)

- People (professionals/staff/family/carers/public) have negative expectations about the person and their behaviour.
- Any behaviour can be interpreted as 'challenging', 'dangerous' or 'risky'.
- Failure to recognise behaviour as legitimate form of communication.
- Risk-averse assessments made about the person.
- Restrictive practices used based on that assessment:
  - liberty restricted
  - access to community and activities restricted
  - over-medication
  - wrong medication used
  - unnecessary physical restraints used.
- Admission to specialist services (sometimes far from home area and family).
- Labels are hard to change, and a person may have that label for the rest if their life and their service provision may reflect that throughout their life, even if it is no longer a relevant label.

Activity 9.4 Reflection (page 141)

- What if the person does not communicate verbally?
- Can we make our communication (of all kinds) accessible and understandable?
- How can we be sure that the person with a learning disability understands what we are telling them?
- Does the person understand the treatment?
- How can we be sure that the person with learning disabilities consents to the treatment?
- How can we be sure that the person will comply with treatment (i.e., take their medication correctly)?
- Does the person need a supporter with them?
- Can the person physically access the service?
- What if the appointment takes too much time?
- What if the person refuses treatment?
- What if the person shows difficult behaviour?

Activity 9.5 Critical thinking (page 143)

Here are some that we thought of. You may have thought of many different ones:

- pull yourself together;
- this coffee is to die for;
- keep an eye out for her;
- has the cat got your tongue?
- let's toast the bride.

Activity 9.6 Critical thinking (page 149)

You may already be familiar with the idea of an 'autism-friendly' environment; some of the things you could consider for any workplace to make it more manageable for a people with hypersensitivity are:

- tidy, neat and clear spaces;
- strong-smelling items locked away/kept separate;
- food eaten in a different space;
- plain colours/lack of 'fussy' patterns in carpets, curtains, etc.;

- visual representations/directions;
- quiet sessions;
- longer appointments.

Activity 9.7 Critical thinking (page 151)

As in a previous discussion point, many of the considerations here will be personal reflections with no 'right or wrong' answers. In terms of lessening the impact of touch for a hypersensitive person, some ideas could be:

- get to know the person (see Mark's advice earlier) and understand exactly what their needs and tolerances are;
- adapt materials you use (bandages, dressings, etc.) to a material or texture that the person can manage;
- explain to the person exactly why something like a dressing is needed;
- let the person use their own pyjamas and clothing as far as possible;
- staff training to enhance understanding of these issues;
- always ask permission before touching the person;
- allow space for the person so that there is unlikely to be accidental touching by other people.

Activity 9.8 Critical thinking (page 153)

As in a previous exercise, some of the answers here will be personal to you and will reflect your own feelings. We would urge you consider this: although some of these interactions may make us feel a little uncomfortable or foolish (and may or may not work) the breakthroughs that can be made with people are significant. Social communication for people with learning disabilities and autism and engaging with another person just for the joy of it can be very challenging so if we have to endure a little embarrassment to help facilitate this, we must put the needs of the person above our own, and engage with this; we hope that you would do the same.

Does it matter that it may not be 'age-appropriate'?

As long-serving Learning Disabilities Nurses, we do believe that age-appropriate interaction is important, as it sends a positive image of people with learning disabilities to the public (and professionals) who often tend to consider people with learning disabilities as being like children, even when they are not, and talk down to them.

It is important that people are given every opportunity to communicate and express themselves, whatever that takes. Taking a more long-term view; if a person can communicate effectively, and we facilitate and respect this, it could offer a chance of a range of communication possibilities that may well develop into more age-appropriate interactions as the person's abilities grow. The key here is to open the channels of communication – how they develop over a longer-term period is secondary at this stage.

Activity 9.9 Critical thinking (page 156)

Who are the key people to work with and why?

- *Billy's parents* as they know him the best and have the most stabilising influence on him.
- They will have been through many changes and similar situations with Billy during his life and will know the strategies that work.
- They may have legal responsibility for him and the decisions made for and about him.
- They will know best how to involve him in decision-making.
- *Billy's brother James,* for most of the same reasons.

- He may see James as a role model; if James will enter the hospital and encourage him, this could be effective.
- Billy respects his opinion and will listen to him.
- *Louise the Community Learning Disabilities Nurse* as this is another positive, stable and long-lasting relationship.
- Louise adds a strong multi-disciplinary aspect to this, and a professional learning disabilities perspective and understanding.

What might you do before the date of the admission?

- The real key here is careful preparation to help Billy to be able to manage the disruption that the hospital visit will cause him.
- One important element will be helping Billy get to know the staff who will work with him by:
  o starting with photographs, show him the people he will meet on the ward (in uniforms if they wear them), with their name, and leave the photos with him so e can become familiar with them over time;
  o identify a small team of key nurses – as many as possible should meet Billy before his admission, in a safe familiar environment;
  o arrange for Billy and his family to make at least one visit to the ward before the admission, preceded by clear photographs of the ward and any areas he will visit while he is there;
  o when he visits arrange for him to meet key people.

How would you use staff during (and before) the admission?

- Staff should meet Billy before his admission.
- Keep as small and regular team as possible.
- Identify key people who will be as constant and present as possible during Billy's stay.
- Make an agreement with catering staff to meet Billy's food and drink preferences.

How might you adjust the environment to suit Billy?

- Private room if possible (if not, as quiet a space as possible on the ward).
- Ensure that decoration in Billy's environment is as plain as possible (incorporating his favourite green colour if possible).
- Have visual representations of key activities and key people.
- Use 'now and next' book to reassure him.
- Use Billy's own pyjamas and Harry Potter bed linen (including weighted blankets as needed).
- Allow space in Billy's environment for him to pace and move around.
- Do whatever you can to limit exposure to strong smells (side room, other people eat away from Billy).
- Allow the use of Billy's favourite Glade plug-in in his room.
- Avoid times when multiple people are in Billy's room whenever possible.
- Allow the use of noise-cancelling headphones.
- Use of Billy's own plates, cups and cutlery, etc. so that he is familiar with them.

What strategies might you use incorporating Billy's interests, and how might these help Billy and you?

- Use any stories and plot lines from Harry Potter that illustrate something like this happening. Not necessarily a hospital visit, but a situation where a key character manages a change in situation and there is a good outcome.
- Create stories with Billy using the Harry Potter characters to demonstrate what could happen. Use of 'What would Harry/Hermione/Ron/Hagrid do in this situation?' scenarios.
- Use watching Harry Potter videos or having a story as rewards for accepting specific situations and activities.
- Allow Billy to decorate his room with posters and pictures of the characters.
- Just engage with Billy about this topic and talk to him about it.

- Learn a bit about it yourself (if you do not know much) so that you can engage positively with him on this topic.

What training and support may staff need?

- Some basic autism-awareness training.
- Give staff the time and support to make the adjustments described above (including the catering staff).

Who might you need to liaise with in the hospital and why?

- Catering staff (dietary needs and the way food should be presented).
- Cleaning staff (avoidance of strong-smelling cleaning products).
- Portering and other support staff so that they are aware of Billy's needs in terms of noise and environment, and not meeting strangers.
- Whole ward team so that they have awareness, even those not working directly with Billy.
- Hospital Learning Disabilities Liaison Nurse to support the whole process.

Annotated further reading

Soderback, I. (2015) *The International Handbook of Occupational Therapy Interventions.* Springer: London.

This book covers occupational therapy and the importance of evidence-based perspectives in occupational therapy intervention.

Useful websites

The video *In My Language* provides a useful insight:

https://www.youtube.com/watch?v=JnylM1hI2jc

This site will provide you with further information on sensory issues:

https://learningdisabilitymatters.co.uk/sensory-information/

This site provides you with insight into the struggles and the risks some families have faced getting reasonable adjustments, and information on training within the NHS:

https://www.olivermcgowan.org/

Chapter 10 Children living with complexity

Introduction

In previous chapters we have discussed the broader context, treatment and experiences of people living with complex needs, including mental health issues. Much of this is transferable to the experiences of children and their families, so we will signpost to the relevant discussions. Now we will focus on the needs of children living with complexity, and their families, discussing capacity, consent and legalities around them for this group. We will explore the models of care and transitions of care.

Definitions

In Chapter 1, we accepted a definition of complex care that noted the mismatch between needs and the system. In Chapter 6, we provided a definition of a child, as someone under eighteen. For children and young people, 'children with medical complexity' includes those with a higher risk for chronic physical, developmental, behavioural, or emotional conditions, and who need access to healthcare beyond the general amount (Cohen et al., 2018). This is taken to mean those with fragile chronic conditions, associated with increased healthcare use and costs. That definition does cover a broad range of groups, all of whom require intensive support and care coordination. Children with complex needs often have challenges, including specialist medical procedures, issues with decision-making and capacity, and the impact on family life (Page et al., 2020). Children from minority groups have more trouble accessing the services they need – an example of intersectionality (Brenner et al., 2018). Race, location, language and culture impacted the access to services, health outcomes and support needs.

Statistics

The *National Service Framework* (Standard 8: Disabled Children and Young People and those with Complex Health Needs) noted a rise in the numbers of children with complex needs, linking it to the increased survival of pre-term babies and children with severe trauma or illnesses such as cerebral palsy, cystic fibrosis and Duchenne muscular dystrophy (Department of Health, 2004; Pinney, 2017).

In 2007, the Department for Education and Skills estimated 100,000 disabled children had complex care needs (Council for Disabled Children and True Colours Trust, 2017). In 2017, this figure increased to 118,000 (Pinney, 2017); much of this increase was around school children with those complex needs, which may be linked to improved identification in the educational system, whereas in social care there were only 2250 children whose support was identified as related to disability. Children with learning disabilities and autistic spectrum disorder make up a considerable number of those with complex needs (Chapter 9). This may reflect the tightening of budgets and access, but equally may be due to the support children are receiving earlier in their journey.

These children are often connected with the health services from birth and are often placed in special schools with additional support (Pinney, 2017). Sometimes planning for their care begins before birth – consider the scenario of Harry, who you have met before in this book, and the preparations his family took prior to his arrival.

Case study: Harry

As a child with haemophilia, Harry's involvement with the health services started before birth, with the need for planning for a safe birth. In fact, for families with genetic disorders or risks it may begin before conception.

This planning included multiple scans to find out his gender and plans for bruising caused by the trauma of birth. In addition, it required the family to consider planning for a child whose needs would add complexity to their lives.

Activity 10.1   Critical thinking

Read the case study above about Harry and his family and then answer the following.

What actions should Harry's parents take prior to his birth to ensure they had support to manage his needs?

Which departments do you think might be involved?

A brief outline answer is provided at the end of the chapter.

Family-centred care

When working with children, it is vital that we are mindful of those around them. We have stressed the emotional and physical fatigue that day-to-day life can bring for those living with complexity (Chapter 8); this is the same for those caring for children with complex needs, with exhaustion as a major issue (Dawood and Price, 2015). There are three main considerations to be mindful of when working with families in this way, particularly with parents or primary caregivers (Page et al., 2020): the level of responsibilities for the parent, the impact on their daily life and their journey across years and lifespan of the child. They may be responsible for major medical treatments, coordination of care, advocating for their families' needs and balancing the needs of their whole family. If they progress from novice to expert, some of that might become commonplace. The deepening of their relationships with key members of staff and teams may improve as time passes.

Brenner et al. (2018) provided some evidence around the impact on the parents' coping skills, the pressure of their responsibilities causing harm to their physical health, financial situation, employment, mental health, social lives and identity. Parents frequently put their children's needs before their own, which often meant that their needs were unmet. Some of them may be reluctant to accept help, perhaps from the cultural pressures of being seen to need help, or they may work hard to ensure a life comparable to a child without these challenges for their own child (Dawood and Price, 2015). But they may find that they aren't welcome in certain public spaces because of behaviours that draw attention (Currie and Szabo, 2019, 2020); this is an issue around public awareness and fear of difference. The stigma of differences, particularly with children who are neuro-divergent, is a clash with the social norms worsened by the invisible nature of the conditions (see Chapter 9). Sometimes this is referred to as intense parenting: the extra effort required of parents of children with complex needs (see Figure 3.1) (Woodgate et al., 2015; Woodgate et al., 2016). Take a moment and just consider what aspects of their lives must be impacted; then, if you want to, you can read more in Woodgate et al.'s paper (2015).

For many families, this may not change as the child grows into an adult and transitions from paediatric services to adult ones.

Although at the stage we discussed in Harry's scenario, the options for care were taken by his parents, working with their healthcare team, later in a child's life, their ability to take ownership of their care grows and develops. Sometimes parental decision-making brings them into conflict with the healthcare team, where their grief around the loss of the child they imagined they would have conflicts with dealing with the reality and planning for the future of the child. This can result in court cases, some of them high profile, such as the Charlie Gard case. Some older children may be able to feed into these decisions as their understanding grows.

Capacity, consent and competence

Competency relates to the right to make autonomous decisions, and in children that depends on the laws of the country of residence (World Health Organization, 2021). You should be aware that the capacity of a child changes: some children can advocate for themselves based on their knowledge and experiences. As they grow, so may their ability to engage in discussions around their choices, but the wishes of a younger child should be heard. The World Health Organization (2021) defines a quality framework for those health services which are 'adolescent-friendly'.

Adolescent-friendly healthcare services: criteria for quality

- **accessible**: *adolescents can obtain the available health services.*
- **acceptable**: *adolescents are willing to obtain the available health services.*
- **equitable**: *all adolescents, not just selected groups, can obtain the available health services.*
- **appropriate**: *the health services are those that adolescents need.*
- **effective**: *the right health services are provided in the right way and make a positive contribution to health.*

(World Health Organization, 2021, p. 6)

Capacity discussions in children often centre around treatment, sexual or reproductive choices. This is no less so in those living with complexity; in fact, they may demonstrate a desire to take ownership of their treatment earlier if they have lived with it a long time. Equally they may disengage, particularly if they have experienced frightening situations with healthcare (Dawood and Price, 2015). Whichever the child feels, you have a duty of care to treat decisions and care with the same ethical principles as you demonstrate in other areas of your practice (Dawood and Price, 2015). Adolescents have the right to express their choices, access the services they need and assert the rights they have (Unicef, 1989).

A principle that can be challenging is around autonomy; although older children may have some autonomy in their choices, there are processes and systems in place to protect and support them (Dawood and Price, 2015). The role of the caregiver or parent is a central one; they can act as care coordinators or case managers, and you need to be mindful of the energies and time invested to do so.

Fraser guidelines

The Fraser guidelines focus on sexual health, where reliable information and access to care is vital for young people (generally defined as fourteen to 24 years of age) (Latham-Cork et al., 2018). This requires that a young person is over thirteen, can understand the advice given and cannot be persuaded to inform their parents with or without support.

Gillick competence

The Gillick competency allows children to make decisions without parental consent if they are deemed able to do so. This arose from case law (House of Lords in Gillick v

West Norfolk and Wisbech AHA [1986]), where the mothers of some girls under sixteen sought to overturn the advice from the Department of Health that doctors could provide contraceptive advice and treatment without parental consent (Griffith, 2021). The child must have two factors to allow them to be deemed Gillick competent: these are maturity and intelligence. Maturity requires that the child have the experience, awareness of the decision itself and capacity to manage the decision-making influences they may experience. Intelligence requires them to understand the decision, have the ability to weigh up risks and benefits and awareness of the longer-term impact of their decisions.

To assess a child for Gillick competence, the healthcare professional should take account of several factors: The child should have:

- an ability to understand that there is a choice, and that the decision has consequences;
- the desire and ability to make that choice, including nominating someone else to make the decision if they wish;
- understanding of the risks and side-effects of the treatment;
- understanding of the options available to them and the risks associated with the alternative treatments;
- understanding of the impact of choosing to have no treatment;
- understanding of the longer-term consequences of the treatment, including impact on schooling, family and welfare;
- freedom from pressure.

In R (Axon v Secretary of State for Health [2006]), a case where the parent challenged the policy of confidentiality for children seeking advice on sexual matters, it was found that the Gillick principles could be more broadly applied to other treatments. Moscati and colleagues highlighted the statutory presumption of capacity for those aged sixteen and over, with the High Court determining that healthcare professionals should involve them where any question over treatment might be raised. These cases demonstrate the inequalities and powers that influence the more vulnerable members of society was well supported with both case law and literature on the topic.

Capacity and children with complex needs

For our group of children, those with complex needs, this may mean that there are times as they develop and grow that their desire to control their treatment becomes more evident, and their right to do so can emerge as a conversation with the child and their family. Although various models of shared decision-making apply to children as well as adults, the WHO have published a practical guideline that holds many useful methods and information (World Health Organization, 2021). It suggests four steps (see Figure 10.1) which support particularly adolescents to move towards a decision with their healthcare team and parents. As you can see, it mirrors other shared decision-making models but adds the issues for young people, which is important to consider.

Overview of practical steps to assess adolescent capacity and support adolescents' autonomous decision-making

This section gives an overview of all steps at a glance. For details, click on the corresponding step.

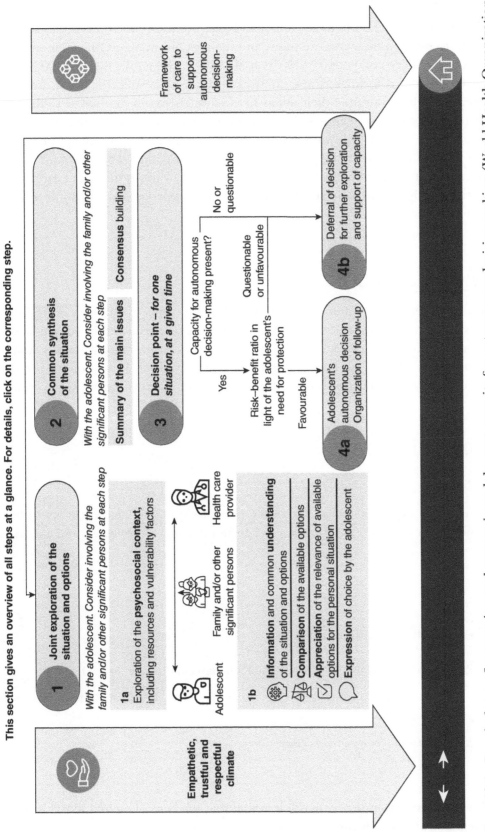

Figure 10.1 Practical steps for assessing and supporting adolescent capacity for autonomous decision-making (World Health Organization, 2021, p. 15)

There is some overlap between moral and legal claims to decision-making as children begin to develop their own opinions and feelings but may not fully demonstrate that they have Gillick competence (Navin et al., 2021). The adults have ethical, moral and legal obligations to work to the child's best interests, especially when their current choices might undermine their ability to have well-being in the future. Children's ability to understand the reality of death or serious illness is often limited. The skill of the practitioner is a key issue within all levels of decision-making in health or social care, but perhaps more so in children who are living with complexity – whether that be the condition or the treatments (Woodman et al., 2018). Various models of care within services that might have contact with children living with complexity exist; we will explore just a few of them.

Models of care

The requirement to commission and plan for the needs of children living with complexity seems obvious, and yet the *National Framework* is criticised by commissioners for a lack of information about the likely demand for continuing care or any supporting information (Pinney, 2017). The organisations involved rely heavily on the information produced by the education sector – transferability of information is a key necessity.

Case study: Harry

To recap …

As a child with haemophilia, Harry's involvement with the health services started before birth, with the concerns his parents had about living in the community with a child with complex long-term needs.

Activity 10.2   Critical thinking

Read the scenario above about Harry and his family and then answer the following.

What MDT might be involved at the earliest stages of Harry's life, including during Rosemary's pregnancy?

A brief outline answer is provided at the end of the chapter.

As you can see from the scenario, it is vital that the care of a child like this should be integrated and coordinated.

Integrated care

The importance of integrated care is, hopefully, clear for you by this stage in the book, with the mismatch between needs and the health and social care system causing major issues for the families (Brenner et al., 2018). So, the necessity for joined-up working across the system becomes obvious, particularly when you link the social and political determinants of health (Chapters 2 and 3). The need for the political desire to make the necessary changes to the system is obvious; advocacy is key in creating that desire, whether that comes from patient groups or healthcare professionals. There is strong evidence that, in creating a better experience and outcomes for these children and their families we save the system money (Cohen et al., 2012). It saves the families' money. Goodwin et al. (2021) provided a list of design features that had a massive impact:

- *personal level:* holistic focus, supporting people to be more functional, independent and resilient, with increased self-management;
- *clinical and service:* multiple referrals into a single point of entry where care coordination can happen. Named care coordinators with continuity;
- *community:* including the local community. Building awareness and trust improves engagement and legitimacy and provides care coordinators with resources;
- *functionality:* the necessity for communication between the team and shared records is key. They suggest a high-touch, low-tech method to improve collaboration and meaningful conversations;
- *organisational:* target the correct service users, localise care coordination and provide leadership and long-term commitments from commissioners;
- *systematic:* integrated health and social care alongside a political narrative that includes holistic care coordination allows long-term planning and stability.

Equally, a lack of planning to measure outcomes has meant that services do not have time to mature before they are asked to provide evidence of their effectiveness.

Care coordination

We discussed care coordination previously (Chapter 5); it is a role that requires considerable skill in relationship building, both with the families and other health or social care teams (Looman et al., 2013).

Transitional care

Transitional care can be included in the broad sweep of definitions since it may be used in relation to transition between acute and community, or child and adult services. The ideal is to provide a set of actions to ensure coordination and continuity of healthcare as patients move between medical teams, locations and levels of care.

To design services that allow adolescents to move into adult services, there are key factors that should be in place, such as named individuals working as care coordinator or key worker and training of the staff in the adult service (Queen's Nursing Institute, 2018). Planning should be an MDT effort, with the family and primary care staff involved.

Transitions may refer to location of services, such as a move from an acute hospital to home; once again, holistic discharge planning that includes their family, MDT and primary care is vital (Campbell et al., 2016). It may also include a transition home between those sites, or a choice by the person (whether they are a young adult or someone with learning disabilities) to live in alternative accommodation such as a shared family home or residential accommodation (such as the Star College). Education and support are an intervention that should be included, as well as consideration of the equipment. Some of this may be more advanced technology.

Self-management

The holistic manner of working with someone to support them in learning to manage their own condition and situation to the best of their ability requires awareness of the demands you are making on someone who may have limited energy or time. For children, you must be mindful of the demands on the parents, siblings and others involved (Lozano and Houtrow, 2018). You can see the ways that modifiable and non-modifiable influences can impact self-management behaviours (Modi et al., 2012), if you think about your own lives: how does your family influence your behaviour? What about your community, or the systems in which you live? Some of these can be modified – can you think which you could change in your lives? Others are less easily changed. These things impact people's willingness to keep to treatments regimes or lifestyle changes.

Technology

Some of this can be supported using technology to keep the child at home rather than hospital; the medical progress of some conditions such as haemophilia has changed the treatment from weeks in hospital to subcutaneous injections fortnightly at home! So mechanical ventilators, IV catheters, tracheostomy tubes, feeding devices, catheters and colostomy bags are all examples of technology you may see at home, preventing those disruptive admissions (Elias and Murphy, 2012). You may see pre-filled pill timers, since lifting just the requirement to remember something is helpful. If a child is in hospital, all these things should be considered in advance; much of this often falls into the role of the occupational therapist, but other specialist healthcare practitioners such as speech and language therapists, specialist nurses, social workers and others may also play a role. Again, the child and the family need to be involved in these decisions and discussions throughout. Training can be a massive task: necessary skills include knowing how to use suction or feeding devices (Elias and Murphy, 2012). But once again, we are asking parents and carers to take on a workload that they may not have capacity to deal with in that moment.

Chapter summary

In this chapter, we have explored the definitions and statistics of children living with complexity. We have discussed capacity and consent issues for children and their families. We have placed the child in the context of the systems they encounter, considering the needs of the whole family in the different models of care. We have hopefully put this through the lens of the child and family experiencing this.

As with all chapters, you should be now placing this new information into the context of your practice, considering where you might come across people living in these situations. Whether you work in the acute sector or community, you will encounter people living with these challenges and your professional duty requires an understanding of how you can best meet their needs and work with them.

Activities: brief outline answers

Activity 10.1 Critical thinking (page 163)

Harry's family explored the services that they needed, linking in with other families in the same situation. They contacted the health visitor, specifically to mitigate accusations of abuse due to the bruising children with haemophilia experience. They worked with the midwife and their GP to ensure that they received the right care. The specialist centre liaised with their local team.

Activity 10.2 Critical thinking (page 168)

Although all of the services in 10.1 are relevant, they also included the other support networks, such as other families, to include them as part of their MDT. They also arranged things such as visits to the childcare and school for educational purposes, training with their family and the local MDT (GP, etc.).

Annotated further reading

World Health Organization (2021) *Assessing and Supporting Adolescents' Capacity for Autonomous Decision-Making in Health Care Settings: A Tool for Health Care Providers. Web Annex: Algorithm for Health Care Providers.* World Health Organization. https://apps.who.int/iris/handle/10665/350193

This explores the algorithm that demonstrates the model in more depth.

NICE (2016) *Transition from Children's to Adult services.* https://www.nice.org.uk/guidance/qs140

This sets the quality standards for transition.

Useful websites

https://www.qni.org.uk/nursing-in-the-community/from-child-to-adult/

The Queen's Nursing Institute (2018) – you can explore the learning resources around transition of care.

https://www.rcn.org.uk/library/subject-guides/children-and-young-people-transition-to-adult-services

Royal College of Nursing (2022) – you can explore the key resources on this page.

References

Abdolrahimi, M. Ghiyasvandian, S., Zakerimoghadam, M. and Ebadi, A. (2017) Therapeutic communication in nursing students: A Walker & Avant concept analysis. *Electronic Physician*, 9(8), 4968–77. https://doi.org/10.19082/4968

Abwao, M., Ittefaq, M., Baines, A. and Liu, P. (2021) 'The disabled community is still waiting for equality': what do users have to say about sexual reproductive health of persons with disabilities in online news comments? *Frontiers in Communication*, 6, 94.

Adomako-Mensah, V., Belloni, A., Blawat, A., De Preux, L., Green, E., Jaccard, A., Preux, L. de, Retat, L., Sassi, F., Thiebault, S. and Webber, L. (2020) *The Health and Social Care Costs of a Selection of Health Conditions and Multi-Morbidities*. London: Public Health England

Ahmedani, B. K. (2011) Mental health stigma: society, individuals, and the profession. *Journal of Social Work Values and Ethics*, 8(2), 4-1–4-16.

Al-Beltagi, M. (2021) Autism medical co-morbidities. *World Journal of Clinical Pediatrics*, 10(3), 15–28.

Alderwick, H., Dunn, P., McKenna, H., Walsh, N. and Ham, C. (2016) *Sustainability and Transformation Plans in the NHS*. London: King's Fund.

All Party Parliamentary Group on Complex Needs and Dual Diagnosis (2014) *Factsheet 1: Complex Needs and Dual Diagnosis*. London: Turning Point.

Alliance Scotland (2016) *Scotland's House of Care Learning Report*. Glasgow: Health and Social Care Alliance Scotland

Alsulamy, N., Lee, A., Thokala, P. and Alessa, T. (2020) What influences the implementation of shared decision-making: an umbrella review. *Patient Education and Counselling*, 103(12), 2400–7. doi: 10.1016/j.pec.2020.08.009

Alvarez-Galvez, J. (2016) Discovering complex interrelationships between socioeconomic status and health in Europe: a case study applying Bayesian networks. *Social Science Research*, 56, 133–43. doi:10.1016/j.ssresearch.2015.12.011

American Psychiatric Association (2022) *Diagnostic and Statistical Manual of Mental Disorders*. 5th edn. Washington: American Psychiatric Association.

Aoki, Y. (2020) Shared decision-making for adults with severe mental illness: a concept analysis. *Japan Journal of Nursing Science*, 17(4). doi:10.1111/jjns.12365

Atherton, H. and Crickmore, D. (eds) (2011) *Learning Disabilities: Towards Inclusion*. London: Elsevier.

Attwood, T. (2007) *The Complete Guide to Asperger's Syndrome*. London: Jessica Kingsley.

Baggs, A. (2007) *In My Language.* Retrieved 5 April 2022 from https://www.youtube.com/watch?v=JnylM1hI2jc

Baker, C. (2021) *Mental Health Statistics (England)* (CBP-06988). London: House of Commons Library.

Barnett, K., Mercer, S. W., Norbury, M., Watt, G., Wyke, S. and Guthrie, B. (2012) Epidemiology of multimorbidity and implications for health care, research, and medical education: a cross-sectional study. *The Lancet*, 380(9836), 37–43. doi:10.1016/s0140-6736(12)60240-2

Baron-Cohen, S., Golan, O. and Ashwin, E. (2009) Can emotion recognition be taught to children with autistic spectrum conditions? *Philosophical Transactions: Biological Sciences*, 364 (1535), 3567–74.

Barr, V., Robinson, S., Marin-Link, B., Underhill, L., Dotts, A., Ravensdale, D. and Salivaras, S. (2003) The expanded chronic care model. *Hospital Quarterly*, 7(1), 73–82.

Barry, A.-M. and Yuill, C. (2016) *Understanding the Sociology of Health: An Introduction.* London: Sage.

Beck, N. S., Kim, D. S. J. and Dunn, L. B. (2021) Ethical issues in psychopharmacology. *Focus, 19(1)*, 53–8. https://doi.org/10.1176/appi.focus.20200043

Bekelman, D. B., Allen, L. A., McBryde, C. F., Hattler, B., Fairclough, D. L., Havranek, E. P., Turvey, C. and Meek, P. M. (2018) Effect of a collaborative care intervention vs usual care on health status of patients with chronic heart failure. *JAMA Internal Medicine*, 178(4), 511. doi:10.1001/jamainternmed.2017.8667

Benedicta, B., Caldwell, P. H. and Scott, K. M. (2020) How parents use, search for and appraise online health information on their child's medical condition: a pilot study. *Journal of Paediatrics and Child Health*, 56(2), 252–8. https://doi.org/10.1111/jpc.14575

Blumenthal-Barby, J., Opel, D. J., Dickert, N. W., Kramer, D. B., Tucker Edmonds, B., Ladin, K., Peek, M. E., Peppercorn, J. and Tilburt, J. (2019) Potential unintended consequences of recent shared decision-making policy initiatives. *Health Affairs*, 38(11), 1876–81.

Bodenheimer, T. and Berry-Millett, R. (2009) *Care Management of Patients with Complex Health Care Needs.* Princeton, NJ: Robert Wood Johnson Foundation.

Boehmer, K. R., Abu Dabrh, A. M., Gionfriddo, M. R., Erwin, P. and Montori, V. M. (2018) Does the chronic care model meet the emerging needs of people living with multimorbidity? A systematic review and thematic synthesis. *PLoS One*, 13(2), e0190852. https://doi.org/10.1371/journal.pone.0190852

Bogdashina, O. (2003) *Sensory Perceptual Issues in Autism and Asperger Syndrome.* London: Jessica Kingsley.

Bolton, D. and Gillett, G. (2019) *The Biopsychosocial Model of Health and Disease: New Philosophical and Scientific Developments.* London: Springer Nature.

Bomhof-Roordink, H., Fischer, M. J., van Duijn-Bakker, N., Baas-Thijssen, M. C., van der Weijden, T., Stiggelbout, A. M. and Pieterse, A. H. (2019) Shared decision-making in oncology: a model based on patients', health care professionals', and researchers' views. *Psycho-oncology*, 28(1), 139–46.

Booth, R and Happé, F. (2010) Hunting with a knife and … fork: examining central coherence in autism, attention deficit/hyperactivity disorder, and typical development with a linguistic task. *Journal of Experimental Child Psychology*, 107(4–5): 377–93.

Bowers, L., Brennan, G., Winship, G. and Theodoridou, C. (2009) Communication skills for nurses and others spending time with people who are very mentally ill. Retrieved from https://www.academia.edu/33457749/Communication_skills_for_nurses_and_others_spending_time_with_people_who_are_very_mentally_ill

Bradley, E., Caldwell, P., Gurney, J., Heath, J., Lightowler, H., Richardson, K. and Swales, J. (2019) *Responsive Communication: Combining Attention to Sensory Issues with Using Body Language (Intensive Interaction) to Interact with Autistic Adults and Children*. London: Pavilion.

Brant, C. C. (1993) Suicide in Canadian Aboriginal peoples: causes and prevention. Royal Commission on Aboriginal Peoples and Canada Communication Group, in National Round Table on Aboriginal Health and Social Issues (Vancouver), *The Path to Healing*. Ottawa: Minister of Supplies and Services.

Brenner, M., Kidston, C., Hilliard, C., Coyne, I., Eustace-Cook, J., Doyle, C., Begley, T. and Barrett, M. J. (2018) Children's complex care needs: a systematic concept analysis of multidisciplinary language. *European Journal of Pediatrics*, 177(11), 1641–52.

Brogan, P., Hasson, F. and McIlfatrick, S. (2018) Shared decision-making at the end of life: a focus group study exploring the perceptions and experiences of multi-disciplinary healthcare professionals working in the home setting. *Palliative Medicine*, 32(1), 123–32.

Brown, P., Zavestoski, S., Mccormick, S., Mayer, B., Morello-Frosch, R. and Gasior Altman, R. (2004) Embodied health movements: new approaches to social movements in health. *Sociology of Health and Illness*, 26(1), 50–80. https://doi.org/10.1111/j.1467-9566.2004.00378.x

Bryant, T. (2013) Policy change and the social determinants of health, in C. Clavier and E. de Leeuw (eds), *Health Promotion and the Policy Process*. Oxford: Oxford University Press, 63–81.

Byrne, B., Alexander, C., Khan, O., Nazroo, J. and Shankley, W. (2020) *Ethnicity, Race and Inequality in the UK: State of the Nation*. London: Policy Press.

Califf, R. M. (2021) Avoiding the coming tsunami of common, chronic disease: what the lessons of the Covid-19 pandemic can teach us. *Circulation*, 143(19), 1831–4.

Camacho, E. M., Davies, L. M., Hann, M., Small, N., Bower, P., Chew-Graham, C., Baguely, C., Gask, L., Dickens, C. M., Lovell, K., Waheed, W., Gibbons, C. J. and Coventry, P. (2018) Long-term clinical and cost-effectiveness of collaborative care (versus usual care) for people with mental–physical multimorbidity: cluster-randomised trial. *British Journal of Psychiatry*, 213(2), 456–63.

Campbell, P., Boyle, A. and Higginson, I. (2017) Should we scrap the target of a maximum four hour wait in emergency departments? *British Medical Journal*, 359.

Campbell, F., Biggs, K., Aldiss, S. K., O'Neill, P. M., Clowes, M., McDonagh, J., While, A. and Gibson, F. (2016) Transition of care for adolescents from paediatric services to adult health services. *Cochrane Database of Systematic Reviews* (4).

Care Quality Commission (2015) *Delivering Cost Effective Care in the NHS.* London: Care Quality Commission.

Carers Trust (2020) *The Triangle of Care for Children and Young People's Mental Health Services.* London: Carers Trust.

Casanova, E. and Casanova, M. (2019) *Defining Autism: A Guide to Brain, Biology, and Behaviour.* London: Jessica Kingsley.

Casanova, M., Frye, R., Gillberg, C. and Casanova, E. (2020) Editorial: co-morbidity and autism spectrum conditions. *Frontiers in Psychiatry*, 11, 1–7.

Challis, D., Chesterman, J., Luckett, R., Stewart, K. and Chessum, R. (2018) *Care Management in Social and Primary Health Care.* https://doi.org/10.4324/9781315185217

Chambers, E. and Coleman, K. (2016) Enablers and barriers for engaged, informed individuals and carers: left wall of the House of Care framework. *British Journal of General Practice*, 66(643), 108–9. https://doi.org/10.3399/bjgp16x683797

Cheng, C., Inder, K. and Chan, S. W.-C. (2019) Patients' experiences of coping with multiple chronic conditions: a meta-ethnography of qualitative work. *International Journal of Mental Health Nursing*, 28(1), 54–70. doi:10.1111/inm.12544

Chouhan, K. and Nazroo, J. (2020) Health inequalities, in B. Byrne, C. Alexander, O. Khan, J. Nazroo and W. Shankley (eds), *Ethnicity, Race and Inequality in the UK.* London: Policy Press, 73–92.

Clarke, G., Pariza, P. and Wolters, A. (2020) The long-term impacts of new care models on hospital use: an evaluation of the Integrated Care Transformation Programme in Mid-Nottinghamshire. Health Foundation.

Coggon, J. (2016) Mental capacity law, autonomy, and best interests: an argument for conceptual and practical clarity in the court of protection. *Medical Law Review*, 24(3), 396–414.

Cohen, E., Berry, J. G., Sanders, L., Schor, E. L. and Wise, P. H. (2018) Status Complexicus? The emergence of pediatric complex care. *Pediatrics*, 141(Supplement 3), S202–S211. https://doi.org/10.1542/peds.2017-1284e

Cohen, E., Lacombe-Duncan, A., Spalding, K., MacInnis, J., Nicholas, D., Narayanan, U. G., Gordon, M., Margolis, I. and Friedman, J. N. (2012) Integrated complex care coordination for children with medical complexity: a mixed-methods evaluation of tertiary care-community collaboration. *BMC Health Services Research*, 12(1), 1–11. https://doi.org/10.1186/1472-6963-12-366

Coleman, E. A. (2003) Falling through the cracks: challenges and opportunities for improving transitional care for persons with continuous complex care needs. *Journal of the American Geriatric Society*, 51(4), 549–55. doi:10.1046/j.1532-5415.2003.51185.x

Correll, C. U., Detraux, J., De Lepeleire, J. and De Hert, M. (2015) Effects of antipsychotics, antidepressants and mood stabilizers on risk for physical diseases in people with schizophrenia, depression and bipolar disorder. *World Psychiatry*, 14(2), 119–36. doi:10.1002/wps.20204

Corrigan, P. W., Druss, B. G. and Perlick, D. A. (2014) The impact of mental illness stigma on seeking and participating in mental health care. *Psychological Science in the Public Interest*, 15(2), 37–70.

Coulter, A., Roberts, S. and Dixon, A. (2013) Delivering Better Services for People with Long-Term Conditions. *Building the House of Care.* London: King's Fund, 1–28.

Coulter, A., Kramer, G., Warren, T. and Salisbury, C. (2016) Building the House of Care for people with long-term conditions: the foundation of the House of Care framework. *British Journal of General Practice*, 66(645), e288–e290. https://doi.org/10.3399/bjgp16x684745

Council for Disabled Children and True Colours Trust (2017) Understanding the needs of disabled children with complex needs or life-limiting conditions Retrieved from https://councilfordisabledchildren.org.uk/resources/all-resources/filter/inclusion-send/understanding-needs-disabled-children-complex-needs

Coyne, I., Amory, A., Kiernan, G. and Gibson, F. (2014) Children's participation in shared decision-making: children, adolescents, parents and healthcare professionals' perspectives and experiences. *European Journal of Oncology Nursing*, 18(3), 273–80. doi:10.1016/j.ejon.2014.01.006

Crisp, N., Brownie, S. and Refsum, C. (2018) Nursing and midwifery: the key to the rapid and cost effective expansion of high quality universal healthcare. *Doha, Qatar, World Innovation Summit for Health*, 1–39.

Currie, G. and Szabo, J. (2019) 'It would be much easier if we were just quiet and disappeared': parents silenced in the experience of caring for children with rare diseases. *Health Expectations*, 22(6), 1251–9.

Currie, G. and Szabo, J. (2020) Social isolation and exclusion: the parents' experience of caring for children with rare neurodevelopmental disorders. *International Journal of Qualitative Studies on Health and Well-Being*, 15(1), 1725362.

Cylus, J., Papanicolas, I. and Smith, P. C. (eds) (2016) *Health System Efficiency: How to Make Measurement Matter for Policy and Management.* Copenhagen: European Observatory on Health Systems and Policies.

Dallimore, D. J., Neukirchinger, B. and Noyes, J. (2018) Why is transition between child and adult services a dangerous time for young people with chronic kidney disease? A mixed-method systematic review. *PLoS One*, 13(8), e0201098. https://doi.org/10.1371/journal.pone.0201098

Dalton-Locke, C., Johnson, S., Harju-Seppänen, J., Lyons, N., Sheridan Rains, L., Stuart, R., Campbell, A., Clark, J., Clifford, A., Courtney, L., Dare, C., Kelly, K., Lynch, C., Mccrone, P., Nairi, S., Newbigging, K., Nyikavaranda, P., Osborn, D., Persaud, K., . . . Lloyd-Evans, B. (2021) Emerging models and trends in mental health crisis care in England: a national investigation of crisis care systems. *BMC Health Services Research*, 21(1). https://doi.org/10.1186/s12913-021-07181-x

Damery, S., Flanagan, S. and Combes, G. (2016) Does integrated care reduce hospital activity for patients with chronic diseases? An umbrella review of systematic reviews. *BMJ Open*, 6(11), e011952. doi:10.1136/bmjopen-2016-011952

Dawes, D. E. (2020) *The Political Determinants of Health.* Baltimore, MD: Johns Hopkins University Press.

Dawood, Z. and Price, J. (2015) Decision making: caring for children with complex needs. *Working Papers in the Health Sciences,* 1(12).

Day, W. and Shaw, R. (2020) When benefit eligibility and patient-led care intersect. Living in the UK with chronic illness: experiences of the work capability assessment. *Journal of Health Psychology,* 135910532095347. doi:10.1177/1359105320953476

Department for Constitutional Affairs (2005) Mental Capacity Act: Code of Practice. London: Stationery Office.

Department for Constitutional Affairs (2014) Care Act. London: Stationery Office.

Department of Health (2001) *Valuing People: A New Strategy for Learning Disability for the 21st Century.* London: Department for Health.

Department of Health (2004) *National Service Framework for Children, Young People and Maternity Services: Disabled Children and Young People and those with Complex Health Needs.* London: Department for Health.

Department of Health (2005) Mental Capacity Act. London: Stationery Office.

Department of Health (2009) *Reference Guide to Consent for Examination or Treatment.* 2nd edn. London: Department of Health.

Department of Health (2012) *Long-term Conditions Compendium of Information.* London: Department of Health.

Department of Health and Social Care (2021a) *The National Strategy for Autistic Children, Young People and Adults: 2021 to 2026.* London: Department of Health and Social Care.

Department of Health and Social Care (2021b) *Working Together to Improve Health and Social Care for All.* London: Stationery Office.

Dickman, N. E. and Chicas, R. (2021) Nursing is never neutral: political determinants of health and systemic marginalization. *Nursing Inquiry,* 28(4), e12408. doi:10.1111/nin.12408

Dieterich, M., Irving, C. B., Bergman, H., Khokhar, M. A., Park, B. and Marshall, M. (2017) Intensive case management for severe mental illness. *Cochrane Database of Systematic Reviews,* 2017(1). https://doi.org/10.1002/14651858.cd007906.pub3

Donnelly, M. (2016) Best interests in the mental capacity act: time to say goodbye? *Medical Law Review,* 24(3), 318–32.

Drummond, M. F., Sculpher, M. J., Claxton, K., Stoddart, G. L. and Torrance, G. W. (2015) *Methods for the Economic Evaluation of Health Care Programmes.* Oxford: Oxford University Press.

Eke, H., Ford, T., Newlove-Delgado, T., Price, A., Young, S., Ani, C., Sayal, K., Lynn, R. M., Paul, M. and Janssens, A. (2020) Transition between child and adult services for young people with attention-deficit hyperactivity disorder (ADHD): findings from a British national surveillance study. *British Journal of Psychiatry,* 217(5), 616–22. https://doi.org/10.1192/bjp.2019.131

Elias, E. R. and Murphy, N. A. (2012) Home care of children and youth with complex health care needs and technology dependencies. *Pediatrics*, 129(5), 996–1005. https://doi.org/10.1542/peds.2012-0606

Elwyn, G. and Vermunt, N. P. C. A. (2020) Goal-Based shared decision-making: developing an integrated model. *Journal of Patient Experience*, 7(5), 688–96.

Elwyn, G., Edwards, A. and Thompson, R. (2016) *Shared Decision-making in Health Care: Achieving Evidence-based Patient Choice.* Oxford: Oxford University Press.

Elwyn, G., Durand, M. A., Song, J., Aarts, J., Barr, P. J., Berger, Z., Cochran, N., Frosch, D., Galasinski, D., Gulbrandsen, P., Han, P. K. J., Härter, M., Kinnersley, P., Lloyd, A., Mishra, M., Perestelo-Perez, L., Scholl, I., Tomori, K., Trevena, L., Witteman, H. O. and Van Der Weijden, T. (2017) A three-talk model for shared decision-making: multistage consultation process. *British Medical Journal*, j4891. doi: 10.1136/bmj.j4891

Emerson, E. (1995), cited in Emerson, E. (2001, 2nd edn) *Challenging Behaviour: Analysis and Intervention in People with Learning Disabilities.* Cambridge: Cambridge University Press.

Emerson, E. and Baines, S. (2010) *Health Inequalities and People with Learning Disabilities in the UK.* Available from: https://strathprints.strath.ac.uk/34862/1/vid_7479_IHaL2010_3HealthInequality2010.pdf

Finkelstein, A., Zhou, A., Taubman, S. and Doyle, J. (2020) Health care hotspotting: a randomized, controlled trial. *New England Journal of Medicine*, 382(2), 152–62. https://doi.org/10.1056/nejmsa1906848

Fletcher-Watson, S. and Happé, F. (2019) *Autism: A New Introduction to Psychological Theory and Current Debate.* London: Routledge.

Forbes, H., Sutton, M., Richardson, G. and Rogers, A. (2016) The determinants of time spent on self-care. *Chronic Illness*, 12(2), 98–115.

Foster, N. E., Hill, J. C., O'Sullivan, P. and Hancock, M. (2013) Stratified models of care. *Best Practice and Research Clinical Rheumatology*, 27(5), 649–61.

Freeman, J. L., Caldwell, P. H., Bennett, P. A. and Scott, K. M. (2018) How adolescents search for and appraise online health information: a systematic review. *Journal of Pediatrics*, 195, 244–55. e241.

Frith, U. (1989) *Autism: Explaining the Enigma.* London: Blackwell.

Frith, U. (2008) *Autism: A Very Short Introduction.* Oxford: Oxford University Press.

Frost, R., Rait, G., Wheatley, A., Wilcock, J., Robinson, L., Harrison Dening, K., Allan, L., Banerjee, S., Manthorpe, J. and Walters, K. (2020) What works in managing complex conditions in older people in primary and community care? A state-of-the-art review. *Health and Social Care in the Community*, 28(6), 1915–27. doi:10.1111/hsc.13085

Furst, M., Salinas-Perez, J. A., Anthens, L., Bagheri, N., Banfield, M., Aloisi, B. and Salvador-Carulla, L. (2018) *The Integrated Mental Health Atlas of the Australian Capital Territory Primary Health Network Region.* https://doi.org/10.13140/RG.2.2.18766.97606

Gabe, J. and Monaghan, L. (2013) *Key Concepts in Medical Sociology.* London: Sage.

Gates, B., Fearns, D. and Welch, J. (2014) *Learning Disabilities Nursing at a Glance.* London: Wiley Blackwell.

Gee, P. M., Greenwood, D. A., Paterniti, D. A., Ward, D. and Miller, L. M. S. (2015) The ehealth enhanced chronic care model: a theory derivation approach. *Journal of Medical Internet Research*, 17(4), e86. https://doi.org/10.2196/jmir.4067

General Medical Council (2020) *Factsheet: Key Legislation and Case Law Relating to Decision Making and Consent.* London: General Medical Council.

Gerbild, H., Larsen, C. M., Rolander, B. and Areskoug-Josefsson, K. (2018) Does a 2-week sexual health in rehabilitation course lead to sustained change in students' attitudes?: a pilot study. *Sexuality and Disability*, 36(4), 417–35.

Gilbody, S. (2006) Collaborative care for depression. *Archives of Internal Medicine*, 166(21), 2314. doi:10.1001/archinte.166.21.2314

Gillespie, A. and Reader, T. W. (2018) Patient-centered insights: using health care complaints to reveal hot spots and blind spots in quality and safety. *Milbank Quarterly*, 96(3), 530–67. https://doi.org/10.1111/1468-0009.12338

Golnik, A., Maccabee-Ryaboy, N., Scal, P., Wey, A. and Gaillard, P. (2012) Shared decision-making: improving care for children with autism. *Intellectual and Developmental Disabilities*, 50(4), 322–31. doi:10.1352/1934-9556-50.4.322

Goodwin, N., Sonola, L., Thiel, V. and Kodner, D. L. (2013) *Co-ordinated Care for People with Complex Chronic Conditions: Key Lessons and Markers for Success.* London: King's Fund/Aetna.

Goodwin, N., Stein, V. and Amelung, V. (2021) What is integrated care?, in V. Amelung, V. Stein, E. Suter, N. Goodwin, E. Nolte and R. Balicer (eds), *Handbook Integrated Care*. London: Springer, 3–25.

Grembowski, D., Schaefer, J., Johnson, K. E., Fischer, H., Moore, S. L., Tai-Seale, M., Ricciardi, R., Fraser, J. R., Miller, D., LeRoy, L. and AHRQ MCC Research Network (2014) A conceptual model of the role of complexity in the care of patients with multiple chronic conditions. *Medical Care*, 52. Retrieved from https://journals.lww.com/lww-medicalcare/Fulltext/2014/03001/A_Conceptual_Model_of_the_Role_of_Complexity_in.5.aspx

Griffith, R. (2021) The right to respect for family life, consent, minors and Gillick competence. *British Journal of Nursing*, 30(17), 1042–3.

Guest, H. (2021) A concept analysis of trauma-informed care. *Nursing Forum*. https://doi.org/10.1111/nuf.12626

Guidry-Grimes, L. (2020) Overcoming obstacles to shared mental health decision-making. *AMA Journal of Ethics*, 22(5), E446–451. doi:10.1001/amajethics.2020.446

Gurney, B. N. (2019) Effects of a writing instructional package for students with moderate intellectual disability. *Electronic Theses and Dissertations.* Paper 3340.

Haemophilia Society (n.d.) *The Contaminated Blood Scandal.* Retrieved from https://haemophilia.org.uk/public-inquiry/the-infected-blood-inquiry/the-contaminated-blood-scandal/

Hardy, S. and Joyce, T. (2009) The Mental Capacity Act: practicalities for health and social care professionals. *Advances in Mental Health and Learning Disabilities*, 3(1), 9–14.

Harrison, C., Britt, H., Miller, G. and Henderson, J. (2014) Examining different measures of multimorbidity, using a large prospective cross-sectional study in Australian general practice. *BMJ Open*, 4(7), e004694-e004694. doi:10.1136/bmjopen-2013-004694

Hart, O. and Eastman, K. (2016) How to support patient-centred care: roof of the House of Care framework. *British Journal of General Practice*, 66(644), 164–5. https://doi.org/10.3399/bjgp16x684229

Hausmann, J. S., Touloumtzis, C., White, M. T., Colbert, J. A. and Gooding, H. C. (2017) Adolescent and young adult use of social media for health and its implications. *Journal of Adolescent Health*, 60(6), 714–19. https://doi.org/10.1016/j.jadohealth.2016.12.025

Health Foundation (2012) Helping people share decision-making, in D. Patel (ed.), *A Review of Evidence Considering Whether Shared Decision Making is Worthwhile*. London: Health Foundation, 78.

Health Foundation (2014a) *Closing the Gap through Changing Relationships: Evaluation*. London: Health Foundation, 74.

Health Foundation (2014b) *Ideas into Action: Person-centred Care in Practice*. London: Health Foundation, 20.

Health Foundation (2021). London: Health Foundation. Retrieved from http://health.org.uk/evidence-hub/money-and-resources/persistent-poverty/relationship-between-living-standards-and-health

Health Service Ombudsman. Retrieved from https://www.ombudsman.org.uk/mental-health

Heslop, P., Blair, P., Fleming, P., Hoghton, M., Marriott, A. and Russ, L. (2013) *Confidential Inquiry into Premature Deaths of People with Learning Disabilities (CIPOLD)*. Bristol: Norah Fry Research Centre.

Hodges , H., Fealko, C. and Soares, N. (2020) Autism spectrum disorder: definition, epidemiology, causes and clinical evaluation. *Translational Pediatrics*, 9, 55–65.

Hoffmann, T. C. and Del Mar, C. (2017) Clinicians' expectations of the benefits and harms of treatments, screening, and tests: a systematic review. *JAMA Internal Medicine*, 177(3), 407–19. doi:10.1001/jamainternmed.2016.8254

Holman, D. and Walker, A. (2020) Understanding unequal ageing: towards a synthesis of intersectionality and life course analyses. *European Journal of Ageing*. doi:10.1007/s10433-020-00582-7

Hope, W. (2012) *The Girl in the Panda Hat*. Self-published.

Horgan, A., O Donovan, M., Manning, F., Doody, R., Savage, E., Dorrity, C., O'Sullivan, H., Goodwin, J., Greaney, S., Biering, P., Bjornsson, E., Bocking, J., Russell, S., Griffin, M., Macgabhann, L., Vaart, K. J., Allon, J., Granerud, A., Hals, E., et al. (2021) 'Meet me where I am': mental health service users' perspectives on the desirable qualities of a mental health nurse. *International Journal of Mental Health Nursing*, 30(1), 136–47. https://doi.org/10.1111/inm.12768

Hubbard, R. and Stone, K. (2018) *The Best Interests Assessor Practice Handbook.* London: Policy Press.

Isobel, S. and Edwards, C. (2017) Using trauma informed care as a nursing model of care in an acute inpatient mental health unit: a practice development process. *International Journal of Mental Health Nursing*, 26(1), 88–94. doi:10.1111/inm.12236

Jahagirdar, D., Kroll, T., Ritchie, K. and Wyke, S. (2012) Using patient reported outcome measures in health services: a qualitative study on including people with low literacy skills and learning disabilities. *BMC Health Services Research*, 12(1), 431. doi:10.1186/1472-6963-12-431

Jayatunga, W., Asaria, M., Belloni, A., George, A., Bourne, T. and Sadique, Z. (2019) Social gradients in health and social care costs: analysis of linked electronic health records in Kent, UK. *Public Health*, 169, 188–94. doi:10.1016/j.puhe.2019.02.007

Jones, W. and Klin, A. (2013) Attention to eyes is present but in decline in 2–6 month old infants later diagnosed with autism. *Nature*, 504 (19), 427–33.

Joseph Rowntree Foundation (2015) *Monitoring Poverty and Social Exclusion.* Retrieved from https://www.jrf.org.uk/mpse-2015/disability

Joseph-Williams, N., Edwards, A. and Elwyn, G. (2014a) Power imbalance prevents shared decision-making. *British Medical Journal*, 348.

Joseph-Williams, N., Elwyn, G. and Edwards, A. (2014b) Knowledge is not power for patients: a systematic review and thematic synthesis of patient-reported barriers and facilitators to shared decision-making. *Patient Education and Counselling*, 94(3), 291–309. doi: 10.1016/j.pec.2013.10.031

Joseph-Williams, N., Lloyd, A., Edwards, A., Stobbart, L., Tomson, D., Macphail, S., Dodd, C., Brain, K., Elwyn, G. and Thomson, R. (2017) Implementing shared decision-making in the NHS: lessons from the MAGIC programme. *British Medical Journal*, j1744. doi:10.1136/bmj.j1744

Kaplan, S. G. and Wheeler, E. G. (1983) Survival skills for working with potentially violent clients. *Social Casework*, 64(6), 339–46.

Karam, M., Chouinard, M.-C., Poitras, M.-E., Couturier, Y., Vedel, I., Grgurevic, N. and Hudon, C. (2021) Nursing care coordination for patients with complex needs in primary healthcare: a scoping review. *International Journal of Integrated Care*, 21(1), 16. https://doi.org/10.5334/ijic.5518

Katon, W. J., Lin, E. H. B., Korff, M., Ciechanowski, P., Ludman, E. J. and Young, B. (2010) Collaborative care for patients with depression and chronic illnesses. *New England Journal of Medicine*, 363. doi:10.1056/NEJMoa1003955

Kendrick, T. (2014) Severe mental illness and the GP quality and outcomes framework. *Trends in Urology and Men's Health*, 5(6), 32–4.

Kingsley, C. and Patel, S. (2017) Patient-reported outcome measures and patient-reported experience measures. *BJA Education*, 17(4), 137–44. doi:10.1093/bjaed/mkw060

Kinnear, D., Morrison, J., Allan, L., Henderson, A., Smiley, E. and Cooper, S.-A. (2018) Prevalence of physical conditions and multimorbidity in a cohort of adults with intellectual disabilities with and without Down syndrome: cross-sectional study. *BMJ Open*, 8(2), e018292.

Knaak, S., Mantler, E. and Szeto, A. (2017) Mental illness-related stigma in healthcare. *Healthcare Management Forum*, 30(2), 111–16. https://doi.org/10.1177/0840470416679413

Koloroutis, M. (2014) The therapeutic use of self: developing three capacities for a more mindful practice. *Creative Nursing*, 20(2), 77–85.

Kotz, J. and Dugdale, P. (2014) The impact of incentives upon integrated care for patients with chronic conditions. *International Journal of Integrated Care*, 14(9).

Kuipers, P., Kendall, E., Ehrlich, C., McIntyre, M., Barber, L., Amsters, D., et al. (2011) *Complexity and Health Care: Health Practitioner Workforce, Services, Roles, Skills and Training to Respond to Patients with Complex Needs.* Brisbane: Queensland Health.

Kuluski, K., Ho, J. W., Hans, P. K. and Nelson, M. L. (2017) Community care for people with complex care needs: bridging the gap between health and social care. *International Journal of Integrated Care*, 17(4). https://doi.org/10.5334/ijic.2944

Kwaitek, E., McKenzie, K. and Loads, D. (2005) Self-awareness and reflection: exploring the 'therapeutic use of self'. *Learning Disability Practice*, 8(3), 27–31.

Lamont, S., Stewart, C. and Chiarella, M. (2019) Capacity and consent: knowledge and practice of legal and healthcare standards. *Nursing Ethics*, 26(1), 71–83.

Latham-Cork, H., Porter, C. and Straw, F. (2018) Sexual health in young people. *Paediatrics and Child Health*, 28(2), 93–9.

Leven, T. (2017) *House of Care Patient Experience Evaluation.* Glasgow: NHS Greater Glasgow and Clyde.

Lin, J. L., Cohen, E. and Sanders, L. M. (2018) Shared decision-making among children with medical complexity: results from a population-based survey. *Journal of Pediatrics*, 192, 216–22. doi:10.1016/j.jpeds.2017.09.001

Looman, W. S., Presler, E., Erickson, M. M., Garwick, A. W., Cady, R. G., Kelly, A. M. and Finkelstein, S. M. (2013) Care coordination for children with complex special health care needs: the value of the advanced practice nurse's enhanced scope of knowledge and practice. *Journal of Pediatric Health Care*, 27(4), 293–303. https://doi.org/10.1016/j.pedhc.2012.03.002

Lopez-Vargas, P., Tong, A., Crowe, S., Alexander, S. I., Caldwell, P. H. Y., Campbell, D. E., et al. (2019) Research priorities for childhood chronic conditions: a workshop report. *Archives of Disease in Childhood*, 104(3), 237–45.

Lozano, P. and Houtrow, A. (2018) Supporting self-management in children and adolescents with complex chronic conditions. *Pediatrics*, 141(Supplement 3), S233–S241.

Lumbreras, B. and López-Pintor, E. (2017) Impact of changes in pill appearance in the adherence to angiotensin receptor blockers and in the blood pressure levels: a retrospective cohort study. *BMJ Open*, 7(3), e012586. doi:10.1136/bmjopen-2016-012586

Lysdahl, K. B. and Hofmann, B. (2016) Complex health care interventions: characteristics relevant for ethical analysis in health technology assessment. *GMS Health Technology Assessment*, 12.

Mackenbach, J. P. (2014) Political determinants of health. *European Journal of Public Health*, 24(1), 2. doi:10.1093/eurpub/ckt183

Mandy, W. and Lai, M. (2017) Towards sex and gender informed autism research. *Autism*, 21(6), 643–5.

Manning, E. and Gagnon, M. (2017) The complex patient: a concept clarification. *Nursing and Health Sciences*, 19(1), 13–21.

Mao, A. Y., Willard-Grace, R., Dubbin, L., Aronson, L., Fernandez, A., Burke, N. J., Finch, J. and Davis, E. (2017) Perspectives of low-income chronically ill patients on complex care management. *Families, Systems, and Health*, 35(4), 399.

Maree, P., Hughes, R., Radford, J., Stankovich, J. and Van Dam, P. J. (2020) Integrating patient complexity into health policy: a conceptual framework. *Australian Health Review*. doi:10.1071/ah19290

Marmot, M. (2020) Health equity in England: the Marmot review 10 years on. *British Medical Journal*, 368.

Marmot, M. (2022) Studying health inequalities has been my life's work: what's about to happen in the UK is unprecedented. *Guardian*. Retrieved from https://www.theguardian.com/commentisfree/2022/apr/08/health-inequalities-uk-poverty-life-death?CMP=share_btn_tw

Masnoon, N., Shakib, S., Kalisch-Ellett, L. and Caughey, G. E. (2017) What is polypharmacy? A systematic review of definitions. *BMC Geriatrics*, 17(1). doi:10.1186/s12877-017-0621-2

Masson, T. (2019) *The Knife Hypothesis, A Companion to Spoon Theory*. Retrieved from https://medium.com/@tilaurin/the-knife-hypothesis-a-companion-to-spoon-theory-d20764c28349

Mathers, N. and Paynton, D. (2016) Rhetoric and reality in person-centred care: introducing the House of Care framework. *British Journal of General Practice*, 66(642), 12–13. https://doi.org/10.3399/bjgp16x683077

May-Benson, T. and Schaaf, R. (2014) Ayres Sensory Integration⁻ intervention, in I. Soderback (ed.), *The International Handbook of Occupational Therapy Interventions*. London: Springer.

McFarland, A. and MacDonald, E. (2019) Role of the nurse in identifying and addressing health inequalities. *Nursing Standard*, 34(4), 37–42. doi:10.7748/ns.2019.e11341

McGrath, M., Low, M. A., Power, E., McCluskey, A. and Lever, S. (2021) Addressing sexuality among people living with chronic disease and disability: a systematic mixed methods review of knowledge, attitudes, and practices of health care professionals. *Archives of Physical Medicine and Rehabilitation*, 102(5), 999–1010.

Medical Research Council (2019) *Developing and Evaluating Complex Interventions*. London: Medical Research Council.

Mencap (2007) *Death by Indifference*. London: Mencap.

Mencap (2012) *Death by Indifference: 74 Deaths and Counting*. London: Mencap.

Mencap (2021) *How Common is Learning Disability in the UK?* Retrieved 24 November 2021, from https://www.mencap.org.uk/learning-disability-explained/research-and-statistics/how-common-learning-disability

Michael, J. (2008) *Healthcare for All.* London: Department of Health.

Michlig, G. J., Westergaard, R. P., Lam, Y., Ahmadi, A., Kirk, G. D., Genz, A., Keruly, J., Hutton, H. and Surkan, P. J. (2018) Avoidance, meaning and grief: psychosocial factors influencing engagement in HIV care. *AIDS Care*, 30(4), 511–17.

Mind (2017) *People with Mental Health Problems Made More Unwell by Benefits System.* Retrieved from https://www.mind.org.uk/news-campaigns/news/people-with-mental-health-problems-made-more-unwell-by-benefits-system/

Miserandino, C. (2003) *The Spoon Theory.* But You Don't Look Sick.com. Retrieved from https://butyoudontlooksick.com/articles/written-by-christine/the-spoon-theory/

Modi, A. C., Pai, A. L., Hommel, K. A., Hood, K. K., Cortina, S., Hilliard, M. E., Guilfoyle, S. M., Gray, W. N. and Drotar, D. (2012) Pediatric self-management: a framework for research, practice, and policy. *Pediatrics*, 129(2), 473–85. https://doi.org/10.1542/peds.2011-1635

Monnette, A., Zhang, Y., Shao, H. and Shi, L. (2018) Concordance of adherence measurement using self-reported adherence questionnaires and medication monitoring devices: an updated review. *Pharmacoeconomics*, 36(1), 17–27.

Monroe, J. (2022) Twitter, 19 January. Available at: https://twitter.com/BootstrapCook/status/1483778776697909252

Montgomery (Appellant) v Lanarkshire Health Board (Respondent) and General Medical Council (Intervener) (2015) UKSC 11, Case Library, 12 King's Bench Walk.

Moscati, M. (2022) Trans* identity does not limit children's capacity: Gillick competence applies to decisions concerning access to puberty blockers too! *Journal of Social Welfare and Family Law*, 1–3.

MS Society (2019) *PIP Fails: How the PIP Process Betrays People with MS.* London: MS Society.

Mulley, A., Trimble, C. and Elwyn, G. (2012) Stop silent misdiagnosis: patients' preferences matter. *British Medical Journal*, 345.

National Autistic Society (2021) *What Is Autism?* Retrieved 15 December 2021 from https://www.autism.org.uk/advice-and-guidance/what-is-autism

National Center for Complex Health and Social Needs (2017) *Blueprint for Complex Care.* Camden, NJ: Camden Coalition of Healthcare Providers.

National Institute for Health and Care Excellence (2015) *Older People with Social Care Needs and Multiple Long-term Conditions.* London: National Institute for Health and Care Excellence.

National Institute for Health and Care Excellence (2018) *Decision-making and Mental Capacity.* London: National Institute for Health and Care Excellence.

National Institute for Health and Care Excellence (2019) *NICE Impact Mental Health.* London: National Institute for Health and Care Excellence.

National Institute for Health and Care Excellence (n.d.) Glossary. Retrieved from https://www.nice.org.uk/glossary

National Institute for Health Research (2021) *Multiple Long-term Conditions (Multimorbidity): Making Sense of the Evidence.* Retrieved from https://evidence.nihr.ac.uk/collection/making-sense-of-the-evidence-multiple-long-term-conditions-multimorbidity/

Navin, M. C., Brummett, A. L. and Wasserman, J. A. (2021) Three kinds of decision-making capacity for refusing medical interventions. *American Journal of Bioethics*, 1–11.

Naylor, C., Taggart, H. and Charles, A. (2017) *Mental Health and New Models of Care: Lessons from the Vanguards.* London: King's Fund.

Naylor, M. D., Shaid, E. C., Carpenter, D., Gass, B., Levine, C., Li, J., Malley, A., Mccauley, K., Nguyen, H. Q., Watson, H., Brock, J., Mittman, B., Jack, B., Mitchell, S., Callicoatte, B., Schall, J. and Williams, M. V. (2017) Components of comprehensive and effective transitional care. *Journal of the American Geriatrics Society*, 65(6), 1119–25. https://doi.org/10.1111/jgs.14782

Nazroo, J. Y., Bhui, K. S. and Rhodes, J. (2020) Where next for understanding race/ethnic inequalities in severe mental illness? Structural, interpersonal and institutional racism. *Sociology of Health and Illness*, 42(2), 262–76. doi:10.1111/1467-9566.13001

Ng, Y. K., Mohamed Shah, N., Loong, L. S., Pee, L. T., M Hidzir, S. A. and Chong, W. W. (2018) Attitudes toward concordance and self-efficacy in decision-making: a cross-sectional study on pharmacist–patient consultations. *Patient Preference and Adherence*, 12, 615–24. doi:10.2147/ppa.s159113

NHS England (2014) *Building and Strengthening Leadership: Leading with Compassion.* London: NHS England. Retrieved from www.england.nhs.uk/wp-content/uploads/2014/12/london-nursing-accessible.pdf

NHS England (2016) *The Five Year Forward View for Mental Health.* London: NHS England, 82.

NHS England (2019a) NHS Long Term Plan. London: NHS England.

NHS England (2019b) *Personal Budgets and Direct Payments.* London: NHS England.

NHS England (2021) *The Improving Access to Psychological Therapies Manual.* London: National Collaborating Centre for Mental Health.

NSPCC (2020) Gillick competency and Fraser guidelines. *NSPCC Learning*, 10 June. Retrieved from https://learning.nspcc.org.uk/child-protection-system/gillick-competence-fraser-guidelines

Nuffield Trust (2021) Do patients feel involved in decisions about their care? *QualityWatch.* Retrieved from https://www.nuffieldtrust.org.uk/resource/do-patients-feel-involved-in-decisions-about-their-care

Nursing and Midwifery Council (2018) *Future Nurse: Standards of Proficiency for Registered Nurses.* London: Nursing and Midwifery Council.

Oliver's Campaign (n.d.) About us. Oliver's Campaign. Retrieved from https://www.olivermcgowan.org/about_us

O'Mahony, D., O'Sullivan, D., Byrne, S., O'Connor, M. N., Ryan, C. and Gallagher, P. (2014) STOPP/START criteria for potentially inappropriate prescribing in older people: version 2. *Age and Ageing*, 44(2), 213–18.

Page, B. F., Hinton, L., Harrop, E. and Vincent, C. (2020) The challenges of caring for children who require complex medical care at home: 'The go between for everyone is the parent and as the parent that's an awful lot of responsibility'. *Health Expectations*, 23(5), 1144–54.

Parliamentary and Health Service Ombudsman (2018) *Maintaining Momentum: Driving Improvements in Mental Health Care*. HC 906. London: House of Commons.

Peart, A., Barton, C., Lewis, V. and Russell, G. (2020) A state-of-the-art review of the experience of care coordination interventions for people living with multimorbidity. *Journal of Clinical Nursing*, 29(9–10), 1445–56. https://doi.org/10.1111/jocn.15206

Peate, I. (2019) A systematic approach to nursing care. *Learning to Care E-Book: The Nurse Associate*, 109.

Peisah, C. (2017) Capacity assessment, in H. Chiu and K. Shulman, *Mental Health and Illness Worldwide: Mental Health and Illness of the Elderly*. London: Springer.

Perera, A. (2008) Can I decide please? The state of children's consent in the UK. *European Journal of Health Law*, 15(4), 411–20.

Perkins, A., Ridler, J., Browes, D., Peryer, G., Notley, C. and Hackmann, C. (2018) Experiencing mental health diagnosis: a systematic review of service user, clinician, and carer perspectives across clinical settings. *Lancet Psychiatry*, 5(9), 747–64.

Pfaff, K. and Markaki, A. (2017) Compassionate collaborative care: an integrative review of quality indicators in end-of-life care. *BMC Palliative Care*, 16(1). doi:10.1186/s12904-017-0246-4

Pinney, A. (2017) *Understanding the Needs of Disabled Children with Complex Needs or Life-Limiting Conditions*. London: Council for Disabled Children.

Pratchett, T. (2013) *Men at Arms* (Vol. 15). London: Random House.

Pritchard, C. and Wallace, M. S. (2011) Comparing the USA, UK and 17 Western countries' efficiency and effectiveness in reducing mortality. *JRSM Short Reports*, 2(7), 1–10. doi:10.1258/shorts.2011.011076

Public Health England (2018) *Severe Mental Illness (SMI) and Physical Health Inequalities: Briefing*. London: Public Health England. Retrieved from https://www.gov.uk/government/publications/severe-mental-illness-smi-physical-health-inequalities/severe-mental-illness-and-physical-health-inequalities-briefing

Queen's Nursing Institute (2018) *Transition of Care Programme Final Report*. London: Queen's Nursing Institute, 16.

Ratzliff, A., Unützer, J., Katon, W. and Stephens, K. A. (2016) *Integrated Care: Creating Effective Mental and Primary Health Care Teams*. Oxford: John Wiley & Sons. http://ebookcentral.proquest.com/lib/uniofglos/detail.action?docID=4322619

Reynolds, R., Dennis, S., Hasan, I., Slewa, J., Chen, W., Tian, D., Bobba, S. and Zwar, N. (2018) A systematic review of chronic disease management interventions in primary care. *BMC Family Practice*, 19(1). https://doi.org/10.1186/s12875-017-0692-3

Rodocanachi-Roidi, M., Isaias, I, Cozzi, F., Grange, F., Scotti, F., Gestra, V., Gandini, A. and Ripamonti, E. (2018) Motor function in Rett syndrome: comparing clinical and parental assessments. *Developmental Medicine and Child Neurology*, 61, 957–63.

Roper, N. (1996) The Roper–Logan–Tierney model: a model in nursing practice, in P. H. Walker and B. M. Neuman, *Blueprint for Use of Nursing Models: Education, Research, Practice, and Administration.* New York: NLN Press, 289–315.

Rose, J. (2018) *Fork Theory.* Retrieved from http://jenrose.com/fork-theory/

Royal College of Nursing (2012) *Making it Work: Shared Decision-making and People with Learning Disabilities.* London: Royal College of Nursing, 16.

Royal College of Nursing (2022) *Children and Young People: Transition to Adult Services.* Royal College of Nursing. Retrieved 10 April 2022 from https://www.rcn.org.uk/library/subject-guides/children-and-young-people-transition-to-adult-services

Royal College of Psychiatrists (2019) *Service Capacity in England.* Retrieved from https://www.rcpsych.ac.uk/improving-care/campaigning-for-better-mental-health-policy/service-capacity-in-england

Royal College of Psychiatrists, British Psychological Society and Royal College of Speech and Language Therapists (2007) *Challenging Behaviour: A Unified Approach. Clinical and Service Guidelines for Supporting People with Learning Disabilities who are at Risk of Receiving Abusive or Restrictive Practice.* Available from: https://www.rcpsych.ac.uk/docs/default-source/improving-care/better-mh-policy/college-reports/college-report-cr144.pdf?sfvrsn=73e437e8_2

Russel, G., Stapely, S., Newlove-Delgado, T., Salmon, A., White, R., Warren, F., Pearson, A. and Ford, T. (2021) Time trends in autism diagnosis over 20 years: a UK population based cohort study. *Journal of Child Psychology and Psychiatry*, 1–9.

Rylaarsdam, L. and Guemez-Gamboa, A. (2019) Genetic causes and modifiers of autistic spectrum disorders. *Frontiers in Cellular Neuroscience*, 13, 1–15.

Safer, J. D., Coleman, E., Feldman, J., Garofalo, R., Hembree, W., Radix, A. and Sevelius, J. (2016) Barriers to healthcare for transgender individuals: current opinion in endocrinology. *Diabetes and Obesity*, 23(2), 168–71. https://doi.org/10.1097/med.0000000000000227

Salway, S., Holman, D., Lee, C., McGowan, V., Ben-Shlomo, Y., Saxena, S. and Nazroo, J. (2020) Transforming the health system for the UK's multiethnic population. *British Medical Journal*, 368.

Sauvage, J. and Ahluwalia, S. (2016) Health and care professionals committed to partnership working: right wall of the House of Care framework. *British Journal of General Practice*, 66(642), 52–3. https://doi.org/10.3399/bjgp16x683389

Sawatzky, R., Kwon, J.-Y., Barclay, R., Chauhan, C., Frank, L., Van Den Hout, W. B., Nielsen, L. K., Nolte, S. and Sprangers, M. A. G. (2021) Implications of response shift for micro-, meso-, and macro-level healthcare decision-making using results of patient-reported outcome measures. *Quality of Life Research*. doi:10.1007/s11136-021-02766-9

Schjødt, I., Johnsen, S. P., Strömberg, A., Kristensen, N. R., and Løgstrup, B. B. (2019) Socioeconomic factors and clinical outcomes among patients with heart failure in a universal health care system. *JACC: Heart Failure*, 7(9), 746–55. doi:10.1016/j.jchf.2019.06.003

Schmidt, E. K., Beining, A., Hand, B. N., Havercamp, S. and Darragh, A. (2021) Healthcare providers' role in providing sexual and reproductive health information to people with intellectual and developmental disabilities: a qualitative study. *Journal of Applied Research in Intellectual Disabilities*. https://doi.org/10.1111/jar.12861

Scope (2019) *The Disability Price Tag 2019 Policy Report.* London: SCOPE.

Scope (2022) *Social Model of Disability.* https://www.scope.org.uk/about-us/social-model-of-disability/

Scottish Government (2020) *Long-term Monitoring of Health Inequalities.* Edinburgh: Scottish Government.

Sheridan Rains, L., Echave, A., Rees, J., Scott, H. R., Lever Taylor, B., Broeckelmann, E., Steare, T., Barnett, P., Cooper, C., Jeynes, T., Russell, J., Oram, S., Rowe, S. and Johnson, S. (2021) Service user experiences of community services for complex emotional needs: a qualitative thematic synthesis. *PLoS One*, 16(4), e0248316. https://doi.org/10.1371/journal.pone.0248316

Soderback, I. (ed.) (2014) *The International Handbook of Occupational Therapy Interventions.* London: Springer.

Soley-Bori, M., Ashworth, M., Bisquera, A., Dodhia, H., Lynch, R., Wang, Y. and Fox-Rushby, J. (2020) Impact of multimorbidity on healthcare costs and utilisation: a systematic review of the UK literature. *British Journal of General Practice*, 71(702), e39–e46.

Stacey, D., Légaré, F., Lewis, K., Barry, M. J., Bennett, C. L., Eden, K. B., Holmes-Rovner, M., Llewellyn-Thomas, H., Lyddiatt, A., Thomson, R., and Trevena, L. (2017) Decision aids for people facing health treatment or screening decisions. *Cochrane Database of Systematic Reviews* (4).

Steuber, P. and Pollard, C. (2018) Building a therapeutic relationship: how much is too much self-disclosure? *International Journal of Caring Services*, 11(2), 651–7.

Stickley, T. (2011) From SOLER to SURETY for effective non-verbal communication. *Nurse Education in Practice*, 11, 395–8.

Sweeney, A., Clement, S., Filson, B. and Kennedy, A. (2016) Trauma-informed mental healthcare in the UK: what is it and how can we further its development? *Mental Health Review Journal*, 21(3), 174–92. https://doi.org/10.1108/mhrj-01-2015-0006

Talbott, E., De Los Reyes, A., Power, T. J., Michel, J. J. and Racz, S. J. (2021) A team-based collaborative care model for youth with attention-deficit hyperactivity disorder in education and health care settings. *Journal of Emotional and Behavioral Disorders*, 29(1), 24–33. doi:10.1177/1063426620949987

Taylor, R. R. (2020) *The Intentional Relationship: Occupational Therapy and Use of Self.* Philadelphia: FA Davis.

The King's Fund (2012) *Long-Term Conditions and Mental Health: The Cost of Co-morbidities.* London: King's Fund.

The King's Fund (2014) *Providing Integrated Care for Older People With Complex Needs: Lessons from Seven International Case Studies.* London: King's Fund.

The King's Fund (2015) *Has the Government put Mental Health on an Equal Footing with Physical Health?* https://www.kingsfund.org.uk/projects/verdict/has-government-put-mental-health-equal-footing-physical-health

The King's Fund (2017) *Mental Health and New Models of Care: Lessons from the Vanguards.* https://www.kingsfund.org.uk/publications/mental-health-new-care-models

The King's Fund (2019a) *Outcomes for Mental Health Services: What Really Matters?* London: King's Fund.

The King's Fund (2019b) *Tackling Poor Health Outcomes: The Role of Trauma-Informed Care.* https://www.kingsfund.org.uk/blog/2019/11/trauma-informed-care

The King's Fund (2021) *NHS Hospital Bed Numbers: Past, Present, Future.* https://www.kingsfund.org.uk/publications/nhs-hospital-bed-numbers

Theis, D. R. Z. and White, M. (2021) Is obesity policy in england fit for purpose? Analysis of government strategies and policies, 1992–2020. *Milbank Quarterly,* 99(1), 126–70. doi:10.1111/1468-0009.12498

Thienemann, F., Sliwa, K. and Rockstroh, J. K. (2013) HIV and the heart: the impact of antiretroviral therapy – a global perspective. *European Heart Journal,* 34(46), 3538–46. doi:10.1093/eurheartj/eht388

Thomas, T. and Forbes, J. (1989) Choice, consent and social work practice. *Practice,* 3(2), 136–47.

Thompson-Lastad, A., Yen, I. H., Fleming, M. D., Van Natta, M., Rubin, S., Shim, J. K. and Burke, N. J. (2017) Defining trauma in complex care management: safety-net providers' perspectives on structural vulnerability and time. *Social Science and Medicine,* 186, 104–12. doi:10.1016/j.socscimed.2017.06.003

Toney-Butler, T. J. and Thayer, J. M. (2020) *Nursing Process.* San Francisco: StatPearls [Internet].

Townsend, B., Strazdins, L., Harris, P., Baum, F. and Friel, S. (2020) Bringing in critical frameworks to investigate agenda-setting for the social determinants of health: lessons from a multiple framework analysis. *Social Science and Medicine,* 250, 112886.

UK Government (2013) *Blood: Contamination.* Retrieved from https://publications.parliament.uk/pa/cm201314/cmhansrd/cm131024/text/131024w0002.htm#131024w0002.htm_spnew1

UK Government (n.d.) *Dismissing Staff.* Retrieved from https://www.gov.uk/dismiss-staff/dismissals-due-to-illness

Unicef (1989) Convention on the Rights of the Child.

Vernon, D., Brown, J. E., Griffiths, E., Nevill, A. M. and Pinkney, M. (2019) Reducing readmission rates through a discharge follow-up service. *Future Hospital Journal,* 6(2), 114–17. doi:10.7861/futurehosp.6-2-114

Wagner, E. H. (1998) Chronic disease management: what will it take to improve care for chronic illness? *Effective Clinical Practice*, 1(1).

Waldron, T., Carr, T., Mcmullen, L., Westhorp, G., Duncan, V., Neufeld, S.-M., Bandura, L.-A. and Groot, G. (2020) Development of a program theory for shared decision-making: a realist synthesis. *BMC Health Services Research*, 20(1). doi:10.1186/s12913-019-4649-1

Walker, S. (2020) Systemic racism: big, black, mad and dangerous in the criminal justice system, in R. Majors, K. Carberry and T. S. Ransaw (eds), *The International Handbook of Black Community Mental Health*. Bingley: Emerald, 41–60. https://doi.org/10.1108/978-1-83909-964-920201004

Warrender, D., Bain, H., Murray, I. and Kennedy, C. (2021) Perspectives of crisis intervention for people diagnosed with 'borderline personality disorder': an integrative review. *Journal of Psychiatric and Mental Health Nursing*, 28(2), 208–36. https://doi.org/10.1111/jpm.12637

Wicks, L. and Mitchell, A. (2010) The adolescent cancer experience: loss of control and benefit finding. *European Journal of Cancer Care*, 19(6), 778–85.

Willcocks, S. G. (2018) Exploring team working and shared leadership in multi-disciplinary cancer care. *Leadership in Health Services*, 31(1), 98–109. https://doi.org/10.1108/lhs-02-2017-0011

Williams, B. C. (2017) The Roper–Logan–Tierney model of nursing. *Nursing2020 Critical Care*, 12(1), 17–20. doi:10.1097/01.CCN.0000508630.55033.1c

Williams, D. (2006) *The Jumbled Jigsaw*. London: Jessica Kingsley.

Wilson, N. J., Lin, Z., Villarosa, A., Lewis, P., Philip, P., Sumar, B. and George, A. (2019) Countering the poor oral health of people with intellectual and developmental disability: a scoping literature review. *BMC Public Health*, 19(1), 1–16.

Woodgate, R. L., Edwards, M., Ripat, J. D., Borton, B. and Rempel, G. (2015) Intense parenting: a qualitative study detailing the experiences of parenting children with complex care needs. *BMC Pediatrics*, 15(1). https://doi.org/10.1186/s12887-015-0514-5

Woodgate, R. L., Edwards, M., Ripat, J. D., Rempel, G. and Johnson, S. F. (2016) Siblings of children with complex care needs: their perspectives and experiences of participating in everyday life. *Child: Care, Health and Development*, 42(4), 504–12. https://doi.org/10.1111/cch.12345

Woodman, E., Roche, S., McArthur, M. and Moore, T. (2018) Child protection practitioners: including children in decision making. *Child and Family Social Work*, 23(3), 475–84.

Working Group on Health Outcomes for Older Persons with Multiple Chronic Conditions (2012) Universal health outcome measures for older persons with multiple chronic conditions. *Journal of the American Geriatrics Society*, 60(12), 2333–41. doi:10.1111/j.1532-5415.2012.04240.x

World Health Organization (2018) International Classification of Diseases for mortality and Morbidity Statistics (11th Revision). https://www.who.int/standards/classifications/classification-of-diseases

World Health Organization (2021) *Assessing and Supporting Adolescents' Capacity for Autonomous Decision-making in Health-care Settings.* Geneva: World Health Organization.

Yazdani, F., Bonsaksen, T., Roberts, D., Hess, K. Y. and Karamali Esmaili, S. (2021) The self-efficacy for therapeutic use of self-questionnaire (SETUS): psychometric properties of the English version. *Irish Journal of Occupational Therapy*, 49(1), 21–7. doi:10.1108/ijot-10-2020-0015

Yen, L., McRae, I. S., Jowsey, T., Gillespie, J., Dugdale, P., Banfield, M., Matthews, P. and Kljakovic, M. (2013) Health work by older people with chronic illness: how much time does it take? *Chronic Illness*, 9(4), 268–82.

Young, A. (2019) Key developments in case law: assessing competence in minors. *Practice Nursing*, 2019(3), 140 -2. doi:10.12968/pnur.2019.30.3.140

Zamanzadeh, V., Valizadeh, L., Tabrizi, F. J., Behshid, M. and Lotfi, M. (2015) Challenges associated with the implementation of the nursing process: a systematic review. *Iranian Journal of Nursing and Midwifery Research*, 20(4), 411.

Zarkowska, E. and Clements, J. (1996) *Problem Behaviour and People with Severe Learning Disabilities.* London: Chapman and Hall.

Zheng, S., Hanchate, A. and Shwartz, M. (2019) One-year costs of medical admissions with and without a 30-day readmission and enhanced risk adjustment. *BMC Health Services Research*, 19(1). doi:10.1186/s12913-019-3983-7

Zisman-Ilani, Y., Chmielowska, M., Dixon, L. B. and Ramon, S. (2021) NICE shared decision-making guidelines and mental health: challenges for research, practice and implementation. *BJPsych Open*, 7(5).

Index

Page numbers followed by *f* indicate figures; those followed by *t* indicate tables.